CONTENTS

W9-AUK-247

Current Clinical Strategies
Critical Care Medicine

Third Edition

Paul D. Chan, M.D.

Matt Brenner, M.D.
Assistant Professor of Medicine
Pulmonary and Critical Care Division
University of California, Irvine

Michael Safani, Pharm. D.
Assistant Clinical Professor
School of Pharmacy
University of California, San Francisco

Cameron Dick, M.D.

Fady G. Kadifa, M.D.

Jeffrey McGovern, M.D.

S. Salman J. Naqvi, M.D., M.Sc.

Theodore Shankel, M.D.

Kirk Voelker, M.D.

Humphrey Wong, M.D.

Division of Pulmonary &
Critical Care Medicine
Department of Medicine
California College of Medicine
University of California, Irvine

Editor's Note

This book is intended to present a concise review of potential therapeutic strategies in the management of critically ill patients. Treatment modalities must be individualized based on the medical condition of each patient. This book is written in a highly condensed format, and it is not possible to describe all potential therapeutic considerations, nor provide a complete description of all procedures and their risks. Physicians are expected to have extensive training and supervision in these areas, and to obtain consultation from appropriate specialists as needed. This book should serve as a guide and an aid in the immediate management of critically ill patients.

Acknowledgments: The authors would like to thank Dr. Donald Mahon, and Dr. Gianna Scannell for their assistance in reviewing this book.

Notice: The reader is advised to consult the drug package insert, and read other references before treating any medical problem, and before using any therapeutic agent. The authors and publisher disclaim any and all liability related to this text. Under no circumstances will this text supervene the experienced, clinical judgement of the treating physician. No liability for errors or omissions exists, expressed or implied.

Current Clinical Strategies Publishing
9550 Warner Ave, Suite 213
Fountain Valley, CA 92708-2822
Phone: 714-965-9400 or 800-331-8227
Fax: 714-965-9401

Printed in USA   ISBN 1-881528-21-9

CARDIOLOGY

ADVANCED CARDIAC LIFE SUPPORT

ALGORITHM FOR EMERGENCY CARDIAC CARE

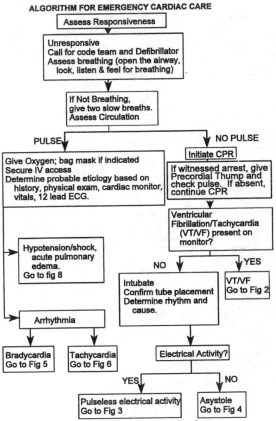

Fig 1 - Algorithm for Adult Emergency Cardiac Care

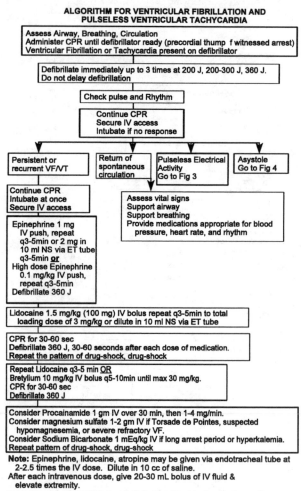

**ALGORITHM FOR VENTRICULAR FIBRILLATION AND
PULSELESS VENTRICULAR TACHYCARDIA**

Assess Airway, Breathing, Circulation
Administer CPR until defibrillator ready (precordial thump f witnessed arrest)
Ventricular Fibrillation or Tachycardia present on defibrillator

Defibrillate immediately up to 3 times at 200 J, 200-300 J, 360 J.
Do not delay defibrillation

Check pulse and Rhythm

Continue CPR
Secure IV access
Intubate if no response

| Persistent or recurrent VF/VT | Return of spontaneous circulation | Pulseless Electrical Activity Go to Fig 3 | Asystole Go to Fig 4 |

Continue CPR
Intubate at once
Secure IV access

Assess vital signs
Support airway
Support breathing
Provide medications appropriate for blood
pressure, heart rate, and rhythm

Epinephrine 1 mg
IV push, repeat
q3-5min or 2 mg in
10 ml NS via ET tube
q3-5min **or**
High dose Epinephrine
0.1 mg/kg IV push,
repeat q3-5min
Defibrillate 360 J

Lidocaine 1.5 mg/kg (100 mg) IV bolus repeat q3-5min to total
loading dose of 3 mg/kg or dilute in 10 ml NS via ET tube

CPR for 30-60 sec
Defibrillate 360 J, 30-60 seconds after each dose of medication.
Repeat the pattern of drug-shock, drug-shock

Repeat Lidocaine q3-5 min **OR**
Bretylium 10 mg/kg IV bolus q5-10min until max 30 mg/kg.
CPR for 30-60 sec
Defibrillate 360 J

Consider Procainamide 1 gm IV over 30 min, then 1-4 mg/min.
Consider magnesium sulfate 1-2 gm IV if Torsade de Pointes, suspected
hypomagnesemia, or severe refractory VF.
Consider Sodium Bicarbonate 1 mEq/kg IV if long arrest period or hyperkalemia.
Repeat pattern of drug-shock, drug-shock

Note: Epinephrine, lidocaine, atropine may be given via endotracheal tube at
2-2.5 times the IV dose. Dilute in 10 cc of saline.
After each intravenous dose, give 20-30 mL bolus of IV fluid &
elevate extremity.

Fig 2 - Ventricular Fibrillation & Pulseless Ventricular Tachycardia

ALGORITHM FOR PULSELESS ELECTRICAL ACTIVITY

Pulseless Electrical Activity Includes:
Electromechanical dissociation (EMD)
Pseudo-EMD
Idioventricular rhythms
Ventricular escape rhythms
Bradyasystolic rhythms
Postdefibrillation idioventricular rhythms

Initiate CPR, secure IV access, intubate, assess pulse.
Doppler ultrasound assessment of blood flow may be useful

↓

Treat Underlying Cause::
Hypoxia (ventilate)
Hypovolemia (infuse volume)
Pericardial tamponade (pericardiocentesis)
Tension pneumothorax (needle decompression)
Pulmonary embolism (thrombectomy, thrombolytics)
Drug overdose with tricyclics, digoxin, beta or calcium blockers
Hyperkalemia or hypokalemia
Acidosis (bicarbonate)
Myocardial infarction (thrombolytics)
Hypothemia (active rewarming)

↓

Epinephrine 1.0 mg IV bolus q3-5 min or high dose
epinephrine 0.1 mg/kg IV push q3-5 min; may give via
ET tube.
Continue CPR

↓

If absolute bradycardia (<60 beats/min) or relative
bradycardia, give atroprine 1 mg IV, q3-5 min, up to total
of 0.04 mg/kg
Consider bicarbonate, 1 mEq/kg IV (1-2 amp, 44 mEq/amp),
if hyperkalemia or other indications.

Fig 3 - Pulseless Electrical Activity

ALGORITHM FOR ASYSTOLE

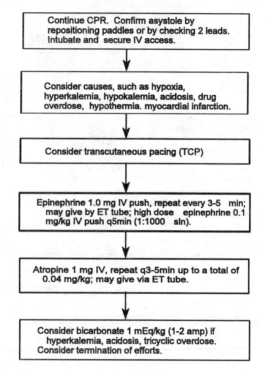

Continue CPR. Confirm asystole by repositioning paddles or by checking 2 leads. Intubate and secure IV access.

Consider causes, such as hypoxia, hyperkalemia, hypokalemia, acidosis, drug overdose, hypothermia. myocardial infarction.

Consider transcutaneous pacing (TCP)

Epinephrine 1.0 mg IV push, repeat every 3-5 min; may give by ET tube; high dose epinephrine 0.1 mg/kg IV push q5min (1:1000 sln).

Atropine 1 mg IV, repeat q3-5min up to a total of 0.04 mg/kg; may give via ET tube.

Consider bicarbonate 1 mEq/kg (1-2 amp) if hyperkalemia, acidosis, tricyclic overdose. Consider termination of efforts.

Fig 4 - Asystole

ALGORITHM FOR BRADYCARDIA

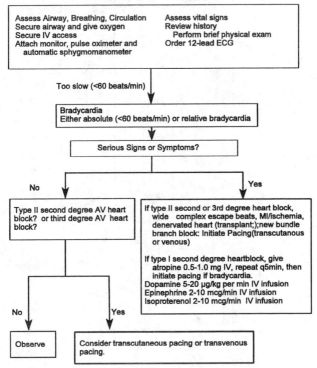

Assess Airway, Breathing, Circulation
Secure airway and give oxygen
Secure IV access
Attach monitor, pulse oximeter and
   automatic sphygmomanometer

Assess vital signs
Review history
   Perform brief physical exam
Order 12-lead ECG

Too slow (<60 beats/min)

Bradycardia
Either absolute (<60 beats/min) or relative bradycardia

Serious Signs or Symptoms?

No

Yes

Type II second degree AV heart block? or third degree AV heart block?

If type II second or 3rd degree heart block, wide   complex escape beats, MI/ischemia, denervated heart (transplant;);new bundle branch block: Initiate Pacing(transcutanous or venous)

If type I second degree heartblock, give atropine 0.5-1.0 mg IV, repeat q5min, then initiate pacing if bradycardia.
Dopamine 5-20 µg/kg per min IV infusion
Epinephrine 2-10 mcg/min IV infusion
Isoproterenol 2-10 mcg/min IV infusion

No

Yes

Observe

Consider transcutaneous pacing or transvenous pacing.

Fig 5 - Bradycardia (with patient not in cardiac arrest).

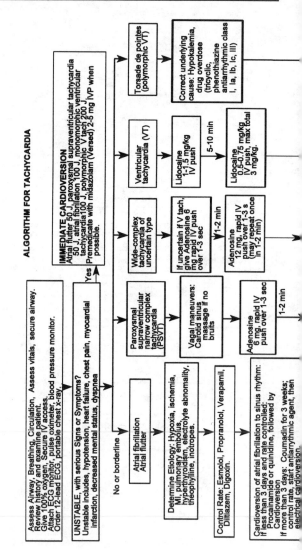

ALGORITHM FOR TACHYCARDIA

Assess Airway, Breathing, Circulation, Assess vitals, secure airway.
Review history and examine patient.
Give 100% oxygen, Secure IV access.
Attach ECG monitor, pulse oximeter, blood pressure monitor.
Order 12-lead ECG, portable chest x-ray.

UNSTABLE, with serious Signs or Symptoms?
Unstable includes, hypotension, heart failure, chest pain, myocardial infarction, decreased mental status, dyspnea

No or borderline → **Yes** →

IMMEDIATE CARDIOVERSION
Atrial flutter 50 J, Paroxysmal supraventricular tachycardia 50 J, atrial fibrillation 100 J, monomorphic ventricular tachycardia 100 J, polymorphic V tach 200 J.
Premedicate with midazolam (Versed) 2-5 mg IVP when possible.

Atrial fibrillation
Atrial flutter

Paroxysmal supraventricular narrow complex tachycardia (PSVT)

Wide-complex tachycardia of uncertain type

Ventricular tachycardia (VT)

Torsade de pointes (polymorphic VT)

Determine Etiology: Hypoxia, ischemia, MI, pulmonary embolus, hyperthyroidism, electrolyte abnormality, theophylline, inotropes.

Vagal maneuvers: Carotid sinus massage if no bruits

If uncertain if V tach, give Adenosine 6 mg rapid IV push over 1-3 sec

Lidocaine 1-1.5 mg/kg IV push

Correct underlying cause: Hypokalemia, drug overdose (tricyclic, phenothiazine antiarrhythmic class I, Ia, Ib, Ic, III)

Control Rate: Esmolol, Propranolol, Verapamil, Diltiazem, Digoxin.

Adenosine 6 mg, rapid IV push over 1-3 sec

Adenosine 12 mg rapid IV push over 1-3 s (may repeat once in 1-2 min)

Lidocaine 0.5-0.75 mg/kg IV push, max total 3 mg/kg.

1-2 min

1-2 min

5-10 min

Cardioversion of atrial fibrillation to sinus rhythm:
If less than 3 days and rate controlled:
Procainamide or quinidine, followed by Cardioversion
If more than 3 days: Coumadin for 3 weeks; control rate, start antiarrhythmic agent, then electrical cardioversion.

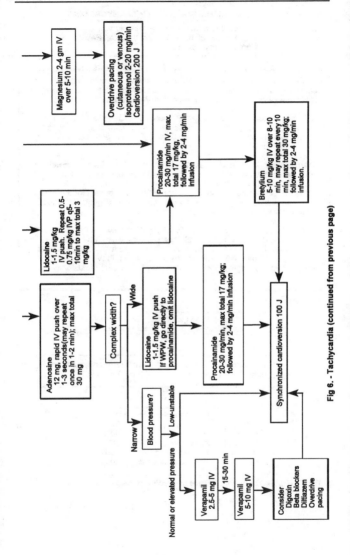

Fig 6. - Tachycardia (continued from previous page)

ALGORITHM FOR STABLE TACHYCARDIA

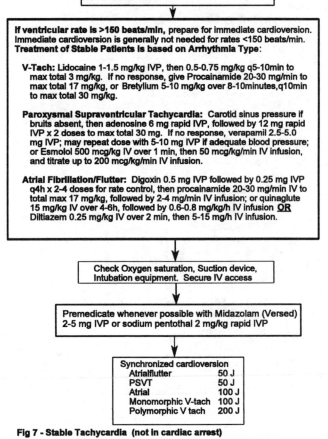

Stable tachycardia with serious signs and symptoms related to the tachycardia. Patient not in cardiac arrest.

If ventricular rate is >150 beats/min, prepare for immediate cardioversion. Immediate cardioversion is generally not needed for rates <150 beats/min. Treatment of Stable Patients is based on Arrhythmia Type:

V-Tach: Lidocaine 1-1.5 mg/kg IVP, then 0.5-0.75 mg/kg q5-10min to max total 3 mg/kg. If no response, give Procainamide 20-30 mg/min to max total 17 mg/kg, or Bretylium 5-10 mg/kg over 8-10minutes,q10min to max total 30 mg/kg.

Paroxysmal Supraventricular Tachycardia: Carotid sinus pressure if bruits absent, then adenosine 6 mg rapid IVP, followed by 12 mg rapid IVP x 2 doses to max total 30 mg. If no response, verapamil 2.5-5.0 mg IVP; may repeat dose with 5-10 mg IVP if adequate blood pressure; or Esmolol 500 mcg/kg IV over 1 min, then 50 mcg/kg/min IV infusion, and titrate up to 200 mcg/kg/min IV infusion.

Atrial Fibrillation/Flutter: Digoxin 0.5 mg IVP followed by 0.25 mg IVP q4h x 2-4 doses for rate control, then procainamide 20-30 mg/min IV to total max 17 mg/kg, followed by 2-4 mg/min IV infusion; or quinaglute 15 mg/kg IV over 4-6h, followed by 0.6-0.8 mg/kg/h IV infusion **OR** Diltiazem 0.25 mg/kg IV over 2 min, then 5-15 mg/h IV infusion.

Check Oxygen saturation, Suction device, Intubation equipment. Secure IV access

Premedicate whenever possible with Midazolam (Versed) 2-5 mg IVP or sodium pentothal 2 mg/kg rapid IVP

Synchronized cardioversion

Atrialflutter	50 J
PSVT	50 J
Atrial	100 J
Monomorphic V-tach	100 J
Polymorphic V tach	200 J

Fig 7 - Stable Tachycardia (not in cardiac arrest)

ALGORITHM FOR HYPOTENSION, SHOCK, AND ACUTE PULMONARY EDEMA

Signs and symptoms of congestive heart failure, acute pulmonary edema.
Assess ABC's, secure airway, administer oxygen; secure IV access. Monitor ECG, pulse oximeter, blood pressure
Check vital signs, review history, and examine patient. Order 12-lead ECG, portable chest X-ray

Determine underlying cause.

Hypovolemia

Administer Fluids, Blood
Consider vasopressors
Apply hemostasis; treat
underlying problem

Pump Failure

Determine blood pressure

Systolic BP <70 mm Hg

Consider
Norepinephrine
0.5-30 µg/min IV or
Dopamine 5-20
µg/kg per min

Systolic BP 70-100 mm Hg

Dopamine 2.5-20 µg/Kg
per min IV (add
norepinephrine if
dopamine is >20 µg/kg
per min)

**Systolic BP >100 mm Hg
and diastolic BP normal**

Dobutamine 2.0-20 µg/kg
per min IV

Consider further Therapy

Diastolic BP >110 mm Hg

If ischemia and hypertension:
Nitroglycerin 10-20 µg/min IV,
and titrate to effect and/or
Nitroprusside 0.1-5.0 µg/kg/min IV

Bradycardia or Tachycardia

Bradycardia
Go to Fig 5

Tachycardia
Go to Fig 6

First-line actions
Furosemide IV 0.5-1.0 mg/kg
Morphine IV 1-3 mg
Nitroglycerin SL 0.4 mg tab
q3-5min x3
Oxygen/intubate as needed

Second-line actions
Nitroglycerin IV (if BP >100 mm Hg): 10-20 mcg/min IV infusion.
Dopamine (if BP <100 mm Hg): 5-20 mcg/kg/min IV infusion.
Dobutamine (if BP >100 mm Hg): 2-15 mcg/kg/min IV infusion
Milrinone: 50 mcg/kg IV over 10 min, then 0.375-0.75 mcg/kg/min IV
infusion

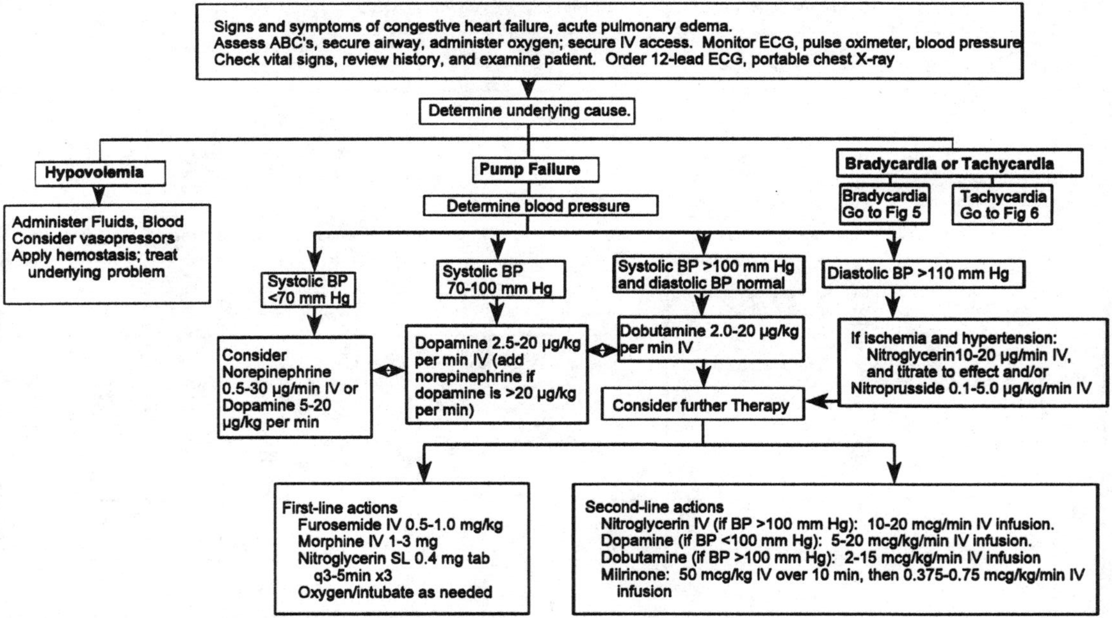

Fig 8 - Hypotension, Shock, and Acute Pulmonary Edema.

ACLS DRUG	DOSAGE	INDICATION	NOTES
INOTROPIC AGENTS: Dopamine	3-15 mcg/Kg/min	Hypotension_septic shock	Dose-dependent pharmacology. correct acidosis prior to use
Dobutamine	2.5-10 mcg/Kg/min	Cardiogenic shock septic shock (concurrent with dopamine)	Monitor CI and SVO_2 to determine optimal dosage. May cause hypotension >15 mcg/Kg/min
Milrinone	50 mcg/Kg IV over 10 min, then 0.375-0.75 mcg/Kg/min IV Infusion	Cardiogenic shock with or without dobutamine	May cause atrial fibrillation, ventricular arrhythmia, thrombocytopenia. hypokalemia.
Digoxin	Patient not previously on digoxin: 0.25-0.5 mg IV, followed by 0.25 mg IV q6h until total dose of 0.75-1.0 mg. Patient previously on digoxin: 0.125-0.25 mg IV may repeat once in 4h. Digoxin Maintenance: 0.125-0.25 mg PO IV qd.	Inotropic support Rate control	When used for rate control, several hours may be required for full effect. Reduce dosage in renal insufficiency. Hypokalemia, hypomagnesemia and hypercalcemia predispose to digoxin toxicity.
Levodopa	250 mg PO qid, increase as tolerated to 1-2 gm/d.		Pyridoxine (vitamin B6) 50 mg PO qd, enhances conversion of levodopa o dopamine peripherally.
Adenosine	6 mg bolus over 3 sec followed by 20 cc saline flush. If no response, repeat 12 mg bolus as above, may repeat x 1: total dose 30 mg.	Paroxysmal Supraventricular tachycardia (PSVT)	Patients taking theophylline, caffeine will not respond. Carbamazepine and dipyridamole will prolong effect. Side effects: chest pain, ectopy, bradycardia, asystole

Atropine	Asystole-1 mg q3-5 min Bradycardia- 0.5-1 mg IV q3-5 min to a total of 3 mg (total 0.04 mg/Kg)	Symptomatic sinus bradycardia. Probably helpful in asystole, and A-V block at the nodal level	Dosage of less than 0.5 mg may be parasympatheticomimetic & further slow heart rate. May cause tachyarrhythmias; use with caution in ischemic heart disease. Possibly harmful in A-V block.
Epinephrine Arrest Dose: Escalating Dose: High Dose: Continuous Infusion:	1 mg IV q3-5 min or 2.5 mg via ET tube 1 mg, 3 mg, 5 mg IV given 3 min apart 0.1 mg/kg IV q3-5 min 30 mg/250 cc D5W at 100 cc/hr, titrate to response	Ventricular fibrillation, tachycardia.	Continuous infusion should be through central venous access. For best absorption deliver via a small bore catheter which extends beyond ET tube and hyperventilate after dose delivered. Dilute ET dose in 10 cc NS.
Isoproterenol	2-10 mcg/min IV infusion	Probably helpful in Torsade de Pointes, and significant bradycardia in denervated hearts. Possibly helpful when used in low doses in symptomatic bradycardia	Not indicated in cardiac arrest or hypotension Possibly harmful when used at high doses for bradycardia
Magnesium	Torsades/VT/VF: 1-2 g Peri-infarction: 1-2 g over 1h, then 0.5-1 g per hour up to 24 hrs	Torsade de Pointes; hypomagnesemia in the perinfarction period.	Monitor for hypotension and asystole. Reduce dose in renal insufficiency.
Calcium Chloride	10% 10 cc/amp =1.0 gm (272 mg elemental Ca) 1 gm IVP or over 5-10 min. replacement: 1 Gm/hr IV infusion	Symptomatic hypocalcemia; myocardial stabilization, hyperkalemia	Monitor for arrhythmias during administration

BASIC CRITICAL CARE PATIENT MANAGEMENT

CRITICAL CARE HISTORY AND PHYSICAL

Chief Complaint: Reason for admission and organ system failure responsible for admission.

History of Present Illness and Hospital Course Prior to Admission to Critical Care Unit:

Diagnostic Studies:

Prior Cardiac History: Angina (stable, unstable, change in frequency). History of myocardial infraction, thrombolytics. History of heart failure; ejection fraction. Call for old EKG's, echocardiogram, stress tests, and catheterization studies.

Chest Pain Characteristics:

1. Pain: Quality of ischemic pain
2. Onset: With activity, awakening from sleep, relation to meals.
3. Severity/Quality: Pressure, tightness, knifelike, pleuritic.
4. Radiation: Jaw, arm.
5. Associated Symptoms: Diaphoresis, dyspnea, back pain, GI symptoms.
6. Duration of episodes.
7. Amelioration: Nitroglycerin, oxygen, rest.
8. Congestive Symptoms: Orthopnea (number of pillows); paroxysmal nocturnal dyspnea, dyspnea on exertion
9. Peripheral Vascular Disease: Claudication, transient ischemic attacks, cerebral vascular accidents; renal disease.
10. Cardiac Risk Factors: Elevated cholesterol or lipids, hypertension; smoking history, male, diabetes mellitus. Family history of atherosclerosis (MI, stroke, peripheral vascular disease - age of onset.) Prior myocardial infarction

Past Medical History: Peptic ulcer disease, COPD. HIV, splenectomy, alcohol, corticosteroids. Functional status prior to hospitalization?

Medications: dosage & frequency. Use of sublingual nitrate.

Social History: Tobacco, alcohol consumption.

Allergies: Dye, aspirin, opiates.

Review of Systems:

PHYSICAL

Vital Signs: T, P, R, BP, Wt, Central venous pulmonary capillary wedge pressure, cardiac output; inputs and outputs.

General: Mental status, Glasgow Coma Scale

HEENT: PERRLA, EOMI

Lungs: Inspection, percussion, palpation, auscultation

Cardiac: Regular rate and rhythm, rubs.

> Cardiac murmurs: 1/6 faint; 2/6 clear ; 3/6 loud; 4/6 palpable; 5/6 heard with stethoscope off the chest; 6/6 heard without stethoscope.

Abdomen: Bowel sounds normoactive, soft-nontender.

Neuro: Deficits in strength, sensation.

> Deep tendon reflexes: 0 - absent; 1 - diminished; 2 - normal; 3 - brisk; 4 - hyperactive clonus.

> Motor Strength: 0 - no contractility; 1 - contractility but no joint motion 2 - motion without gravity; 3 - barely against gravity; 4 - some resistance; 5 -motion against full resistance (normal).

Extremities: Cyanosis, clubbing, edema, peripheral pulses 2+.

Skin: Capillary refill and turgor.

Labs: CBC, PT/PTT; Chem 6, Chem 12, Mg, pH/pCO2/pO2

> CXR, EKG, other diagnostic studies.

Impression/Problem list: Discuss diagnosis and plan for each problem by system.

> **Neuro:** List and discuss neurologic problems

> **Pulmonary:** Ventilator management

> **GI:** H2 blockers, nasogastric tubes.

> **GU/electrolytes-fluid status:** IV fluids, electrolyte therapy.

> **Heme:** Blood or blood products

> **ID:** Antibiotic therapy

> **Endocrine/Nutrition:** Parenteral or enteral nutrition

Admission Check List:

1. **Call for old chart, EKG, and X-rays.**
2. **Stat labs** - CBC, Chem 7, PT, PTT, T&S, ABG, UA.
3. **Additional labs** - Toxicology screens and drug levels.
4. **Additional cultures** - Blood culture x 2, Urine and sputum culture before starting antibiotics.
5. **CXR, EKG**, additional diagnostic studies.
6. **Discuss Case** with resident, attending or fellow, and family.

CRITICAL CARE PROGRESS NOTE

ICU Day Number:
Antibiotic Day Number:
Subjective: Patient is awake and alert
Objective: T max, T, P, R, BP, 24 hr input and output, pulmonary artery pressure, pulmonary capillary wedge pressure, cardiac output
Lungs: Clear bilaterally
Cardiac: Regular rate and rhythm, no murmur, no rubs.
Abdomen: Bowel sounds normoactive, soft-nontender.
Neuro: No local deficits in strength, sensation.
Extremities: No cyanosis, clubbing, edema, peripheral pulses 2+.
Labs: WBC, CBC, ABG, Chem 7.
EKG:
CXR:
Impression/Plan: Overview impression and then discuss by organ system:
    Fluids/Electrolytes:
    Pulmonary:
    Cardiovascular:
    Infectious:
    Endocrine:
    Nutrition:

FLUIDS AND ELECTROLYTES

<u>Maintenance Fluids Guidelines:</u>
    70 kg Male: D5 1/4 NS with 20 mEq KCl/liter at 125 mL/hr.
<u>Specific Replacement Fluids for Specific Losses:</u>
    Gastric (nasogastric tube, emesis): D5 ½ NS with 20 mEq/liter KCL.
    Diarrhea: D5LR with 15 mEq/liter KCl. Provide approximately 1 liter replacement for each 1 kg or 2.2 lb of body weight lost.
    Bile: D5LR with 25 mEq/liter (½ amp) of HCO_3.
    Pancreatic: D5LR with 50 mEq/liter (1 amp) HCO_3.

BLOOD COMPONENT THERAPY

Estimation of Blood Volume:
Total blood volume (TBV in liters) = 7% of body weight in kilograms.

Male = 77 x body weight (kg) = TBV (mLs)

Female = 67 x body weight (kg) = TBV (mLs)

Plasma volume = TBV-(TBV x hematocrit)

Colloid Solution Therapy: Indicated for volume expansion.

Albumin (5% or 25%), useful for hypovolemia and hypoproteinemia; or to induce diuresis with furosemide in hypervolemic, hypoproteinemic patients.

Plasma protein fraction 5% (plasmanate): Contains 130-160 mEq Na/L; indicated for volume expansion.

Hetastarch (Hespan): Synthetic colloid; 6% hetastarch in saline. Similar indications as for albumin.

Crystalloids Solutions: Normal saline, lactated Ringers solution; used for acute volume replacement. 3 cc crystalloid = 1 cc whole blood.

Guidelines for Red Blood Cell Transfusions for Acute Blood Loss:

1. Used to control hemorrhage and replace losses with crystalloids until packed red blood cells are available.
2. If crystalloids fail to produce hemodynamic stability after more than 2 liters administered, give packed red blood cells.
3. If volume replacement and hemostasis stabilize hemodynamic status, wait for formal type and cross match for blood. Otherwise, administer O⁻ negative, low titer blood or type specific (ABO matched), Rh compatible blood which can be prepared in 10 minutes and is not crossed matched.

Guidelines for Blood Transfusion in Acute Anemia:

Consider blood transfusion when hemoglobin is <8.0 and hematocrit <24%, unless patient has symptoms such as chest pain, dyspnea, sepsis, mental status changes. Consider rate of fall in hemoglobin, absolute level of hemoglobin, active bleeding diathesis, underlying coagulopathy, preexisting coronary artery disease or ischemia.

Blood Component Products:

Packed Red Blood Cells (PRBC's): Each unit provides approximately 250 cc of volume, and each unit should raise hemoglobin by 1 gm/dL and hematocrit by 3%. PRBC's are usually requested in increments of two units.

Type and Screen: Blood is tested for A, B, and Rh antigens and antibodies to donor erythrocytes. If blood products are required the blood can be rapidly prepared by blood bank.

Type and Cross Match: Sets aside specific units of donor packed red blood cells. If blood is expected to be needed on an urgent basis, then type and cross should be requested.

Platelets: Indicated for bleeding due to thrombocytopenia or thrombopathy in the setting of uncontrolled bleeding. Each unit of platelet concentrate should raise platelet count by 5,000-10,000. Usual transfused 8-10 units at a time and should increase platelet count by 40-60,000.

Thrombocytopenia Evaluation: Prior to platelet transfusion, the etiology and reversible causes of thrombocytopenia should be evaluated, i.e. decreased marrow production, sequestration, or accelerated destruction. Examine peripheral blood smear; consider of bone marrow biopsy, assess splenic size, and review of all medications that could cause thrombocytopenia.

Fresh Frozen Plasma (FFP): Used for active bleeding secondary to liver disease; warfarin overdose, dilutional coagulopathy (from multiple blood transfusions); disseminated intravascular coagulopathy; vitamin K and coagulation factor deficiencies. Requires ABO typing, but not cross matching.

    a. Components-Each unit contains all coagulation factors in normal concentration, including the labile coagulation factors (V, VIII).

    b. Transfusion Replacement-FFP dosage may be estimated as 8-10 mL/kg. Each unit of FFP contains 200-280 mL, therefore, 4-6 units are usually required for therapeutic intervention. The frequency of dosing depends on clinical response.

Cryoprecipitate:

    a. Indicated in patients with Hemophilia A, von Willebrand's disease, and any state of hypofibrinogenemia requiring replacement (DIC), or reversal of thrombolytic therapy.

    b. Components-Factor VIII, fibrinogen, von Willebrand factor.

    c. Transfusion Replacement-The goal of therapy is to maintain the fibrinogen level above 100 mL/dL. This is usually achieved with 2-4 units/10 kg or 1-2 units/10 kg depending on whether the fibrinogen content in the precipitate is high or low respectively.

PARENTERAL NUTRITION

Peripheral Parenteral Supplementation:

-3% amino acid sln (ProCalamine) up to 3 L/d at 125 cc/h **OR**

-Combine 500 mL Amino acid solution 7% or 10% (Aminosyn) & 500 mL 20% dextrose & electrolyte additive and infuse at up to 100 cc/hr in parallel with:

-Intralipid 10% or 20% at 1 mL/min for 15 min (test dose); if no adverse reactions, infuse 500 mL/d at up to 100 mL/hr.

-Draw blood 6h after end of infusion for triglyceride.

Central Parenteral Nutrition:

-Infuse 40-50 mL/h of amino acid-dextrose solution in the first 24h; increase daily by 40 mL/hr increments until providing 1.3-2 x basal energy requirement & 1.2-1.7 gm protein/kg/d (see formula page 146).

Standard solution: (adjust TPN as needed to maintain normal electrolytes depending on clinical condition of patient)

Amino acid sln (Aminosyn) 7-10%	500 mL
Dextrose 40-70%	500 mL
Sodium	35 mEq
Potassium	36 mEq
Chloride	35 mEq
Calcium	4.5 mEq
Phosphate	9 mMol
Magnesium	8.0 mEq
Acetate	82-104 mEq
Multi-Trace Element Formula	1 mL/d
Regular insulin (if indicated)	10-60 U/L
Multivitamin(12)(2 amp)	10 mL/d
Vitamin K (in solution, SQ, IM)	10 mg/week
Vitamin B12	1000 µg/week

Fat Emulsion:

Intralipid 20% 500 mL/d IVPB infuse in parallel with standard solution at 1 mL/min x 15 min; if no adverse reactions, increase to 100 mL/hr. Serum triglyceride 6h after end of infusion (maintain <200 mg/dL). May use fat emulsion as source of calorie and/or to prevent free fatty acid deficiency.

Cyclic TPN: 12h night schedule; Taper continuous infusion in morning by reducing rate to half original rate for 1 hour. Further reduce rate by half for an additional hr; then discontinue. Finger stick glucose q2h; Restart TPN in afternoon. Taper in beginning & end of cycle; Final rate of 185 mL/hr for 9-10h with 2h of taper at each end for total of 2000 mL.

Special Medications:

-Cimetidine 300 mg IV q6-8h or in TPN **OR**

-Ranitidine 50 mg IV q6-8h.

-Insulin sliding scale.

Labs:

Baseline: Draw labs below. CXR, plain film for tube placement

Daily Labs: SMA7, osmolality, CBC, cholesterol, triglyceride (6 h after end of infusion), urine glucose & specific gravity, phos, Mg, Ca.

Weekly Labs when indicated: Protein, iron, TIBC, transferrin, PT/PTT, zinc, copper, B12, Folate, 24h urine nitrogen & creatinine. Pre-albumin, retinol-binding protein, albumin, total protein, SGOT, SGPT, GGT, alk phos, LDH, amylase, total bilirubin.

ENTERAL NUTRITION

General Measures: Daily weights, I&O. Nasoduodenal feeding tube. Head of bed at 30 degrees while enteral feeding & 2 hours after completion. Finger stick glucose qid, record bowel movements. Consider nutrition consult.

Enteral Bolus Feeding: Give 50-100 ml of enteral solution (ex: Osmolite, Pulmocare, Jevity) q3h initially. Increase amount in 50 ml steps to max of 250-300 ml q3-4h; 30 kcal of nonprotein calories/d & 1.5 gm protein/kg/d. Before each feeding measure residual volume, and delay feeding by 1h if >100 ml. Flush tube with 100 cc of water after each bolus.

Continuous Enteral Infusion: Initial enteral solution (Osmolite, Pulmocare, Jevity) 30 ml/hr. Measure residual volume q1h x 12h then tid; hold feeding for 1h if >100 ml. Increase rate by 25-50 ml/hr at 24 hr intervals as tolerated until final rate of 50-100 ml/hr (1 Cal/ml) as tolerated. 3 Tablespoons of protein powder (Promix) may be added to each 500 cc of solution. Flush tube with 100 cc water q8h. Consider consultation with a nutritionist if long-term enteral nutrition.

Special Medications:

- -Metoclopramide (Reglan) 10-20 mg PO, IM, IV, or in J tube q6h.
- -Cimetidine 300 mg PO tid-qid or 37.5-100 mg/h IV or 300 mg IV q6-8h or in TPN **OR**
- -Ranitidine 50 mg IV q6-8h or 150 mg PO bid or in TPN.

Symptomatic Medications:

- -Loperamide (Imodium) 2-4 mg PO/J-tube q6h, max 16 mg/d prn **OR**
- -Diphenoxylate/atropine (Lomotil) 1-2 tabs or 5-10 mL (2.5 mg/5 mLs) PO/J-tube q4-6h prn, max 12 tabs/d **OR**
- -Codeine sulfate 30 mg PO or in J-tube q6h.
- -Kaopectate 30 cc PO or in J-tube q8h.

RADIOGRAPHIC EVALUATION OF COMMON INTERVENTIONS

<u>Central Intravenous Lines:</u>

Central venous catheters should be located well above the right atrium, and not in a neck vein. Rule out pneumothorax by checking that the lung markings extend completely to the rib cages on both sides. An upright, expiratory x-ray may be helpful. Examine for hydropericardium ("water bottle" sign, mediastinal widening).

Pulmonary artery catheters should be located centrally and posteriorly, and not more than 3-5 cm from midline.

<u>Endotracheal Tubes:</u> Verify that the tube is located 3 cm below the vocal cords and 2-4 cm above the carina; the tip of tube should be at the level of aortic arch.

<u>Tracheostomy:</u> Verify by chest x-ray that the tube is located half the distance from the stoma to the carina; the tube should be parallel to the long axis of the trachea. The tube should be approximately 2/3 of width of trachea; the cuff should not cause bulging of the trachea walls. Check for subcutaneous air in the neck tissue and for mediastinal widening secondary to air leakage.

<u>Nasogastric Tubes:</u> Verify that the tube is in the stomach and not coiled in the esophagus or trachea. Tip of the tube should not be near gastroesophageal junction.

<u>Chest Tubes:</u> A chest tube for pneumothorax drainage should be superior, near level of the third intercostal space. To drain a free flowing pleural effusion, the tube should be located inferior-posteriorly, at or about the level of the eighth intercostal space. Verify that the side port of the tube is within the chest.

<u>Mechanical Ventilation:</u> Obtain a chest x-ray to rule out pneumothorax, subcutaneous emphysema, pneumomediastinum or subpleural air cysts. Infiltrates may diminish or disappear due to increased aeration of the affected lung lobe.

ARTERIAL LINE PLACEMENT

<u>Procedure:</u>

1. Obtain a 20 gauge 1½-2 inch catheter over needle assembly (Angiocath); arterial line setup (transducer, tubing and pressure bag containing heparinized saline), armboard, sterile dressing, lidocaine, 3 cc syringe, 25 gauge needle, 3-0 silk.

2. The radial artery is the most frequently used artery; use Allen test to verify patency of the radial and ulnar arteries. Place the extremity on an armboard with a gauze roll behind the wrist to maintain hyperextension.

3. Prep with providone-iodine and drape; infiltrate 1% lidocaine using a 25 gauge needle. Choose site where the artery appears most superficial and distal.
4. Palpate the artery with the left hand, and use other hand to advance the 20 gauge catheter-over-needle assembly into the artery at a 30 degree angle to the skin. When flash of blood is seen, hold the needle in place and advance the catheter into the artery; occlude the artery with manual pressure while the pressure tubing is connected.
5. Needle and guide-wire kits may also be used; Advance the guide-wire into the artery, and pass the catheter over the guide-wire.
6. Suture catheter in place with 3-0 silk and apply dressing.

CENTRAL VENUS CATHETERIZATION

Indications for Central Venus Catheter Cannulation: Monitoring of central venous pressures in shock or heart failure; management of fluid status; insertion of transvenous pacemaker; administration of total parenteral nutrition, administration of vesicants (chemotherapeutic agents).

Location: Internal jugular approach is contraindicated in patients with carotid bruit, stenosis, or aneurysm. Subclavian approach has increased risk in patients with emphysema or bullae. The external jugular or internal jugular approach may be preferable in patients with coagulopathy, thrombocytopenia. In patients with unilateral lung pathology or a chest tube already in places, consider preferential placement of the catheter on the side of predominant pathology or the side with the chest tube.

Technique of Insertion for External Jugular Vein Catheter:

1. The external jugular vein extends from angle of mandible to behind the middle of clavicle where it joins with the subclavian vein. Place patient in Trendelenburg's position. Cleanse skin with Betadine-iodine solution; using sterile technique, inject 1% lidocaine to produce a skin weal. Apply digital pressure to the external jugular vein above clavicle to distend vein.
2. With an 18-gauge thin wall needle, advance the needle into the vein. Then pass a J-guide wire through the needle; the wire should advance without resistance. Remove the needle, maintaining control over the guide wire at all times. Nick the skin with a No. 11 scalpel blade.
3. With guide wire in place, pass the central catheter over the wire and remove the guide wire after the catheter is in place. Cover catheter hub with finger to prevent air embolization.
4. Attach a syringe to the catheter hub and ensure that there is free back-flow of dark venous blood. Attach the catheter to intravenous infusion.
5. Secure the catheter in place with 2-0 silk suture and tape. The catheter should be removed and changed within 3-4 days. Consider use of

antibacterial coated catheters or "cuffs" in patients with limited access sites or high risks for infection.

6. Obtain a CXR to confirm position and rule out pneumothorax.

Internal Jugular Vein Cannulation:

The internal jugular vein is positioned behind the sternocleidomastoid muscle lateral to the carotid artery (for the "middle approach"). The catheter should be placed at a location at the upper confluence of the two bellies of sternocleidomastoid, at the level of cricoid cartilage.

1. Place the patient in Trendelenburg's position and turn the patient's head to the contralateral side.

2. Choose a location on the right or left. If all other factors are equal (symmetrical lung function, no chest tubes in place), the right side is preferred because of the direct path to the superior vena cava. Prepare the skin with Betadine solution using sterile technique and drape. Infiltrate the skin and deeper tissues with 1% lidocaine.

3. Palpate the carotid artery. Using a 22-gauge scout needle and syringe, direct the needle toward the nipple at a 30 degree angle to the neck. While aspirating, advance the needle until the vein is located and blood back flows into the syringe.

4. Remove the scout needle and advance an 18-gauge, thin wall catheter-over-needle with an attached syringe along the same path as the scout needle. When back flow of blood is noted into syringe, advance the catheter into the vein. Remove the needle and confirm back flow of blood through the catheter and into the syringe. Remove syringe and use a finger to cover the catheter hub with finger to prevent air embolization.

5. With the 16-gauge catheter in position, advance a 0.89 mm x 45 cm spring guide wire through the catheter. The guide wire should advance easily without resistance.

6. With the guide wire in position remove the catheter and use a No. 11 scalpel blade to nick the skin.

7. Place central vein catheter over the wire, holding the wire secure at all times. Pass the catheter into the vein, and suture the catheter with O silk suture, tape, and connect to IV infusion.

8. Obtain CXR to rule out pneumothorax and confirm position.

Subclavian Vein Cannulation:

The subclavian vein is located in the angle form by the medial 1/3 of clavicle and the first rib.

1. Position the patient supine with a rolled towel located between the patient's scapulae, and turn the head towards the contralateral side. Prepare the area with Betadine iodine solution and, using sterile technique, drape the area and infiltrate 1% lidocaine into the skin and tissues.

2. With a 16-gauge catheter-over-needle with syringe attached, puncture the mid-point of the clavicle until the clavicle bone and needle come in contact.

3. Slowly probe down with the needle until the needle slips under the clavicle, and advance slowly towards the vein until the catheter needle enters the vein, and a back flow of venous blood enters the syringe. Remove the syringe, and cover the catheter hub with finger to prevent air embolization.

4. With the 16-gauge catheter in position, advance a 0.89 mm x 45 cm spring guide wire through the catheter. The guide wire should advance easily without resistance.

5. With the guide wire in position, remove the catheter and use a No. 11 scalpel blade to nick the skin.

6. Place the central line catheter over the wire, holding the wire secure at all times. Pass the catheter into the vein, and suture the catheter with 2-0 silk suture, tape, and connect to IV infusion.

7. Obtain CXR to confirm position & rule out pneumothorax.

PULMONARY ARTERY CATHETERIZATION

Procedure:

1. Using sterile technique, cannulate a vein using the technique above, such as the subclavian vein or internal jugular vein.

2. Advance a guide wire through the cannula, and remove the cannula. Nick the skin with a number 11 scalpel blade adjacent to the guide wire, and pass a number 8 French introducer over the wire into the vein. Connect introducer to an IV fluid infusion, and suture with 2-0 silk.

3. Pass the proximal end of the pulmonary artery catheter (Swan Ganz) to an assistant for connection to a continuous flush transducer system.

4. Flush the distal and proximal ports with heparin solution, remove all bubbles, and check balloon integrity by inflating 2 cc of air. Check pressure transducer by quickly moving the distal tip and watching monitor for response.

5. Pass the catheter through the introducer into the vein, then inflate the balloon with 0.8-1.0 cc of air, and advance the catheter until the balloon is in or near the right atrium.

6. As a general guideline, the correct distance to the entrance of the right atrium is determined from the site of insertion:

> Right antecubital fossa: 35-40 cm
> Left Antecubital fossa: 45-50 cm.
> Right internal jugular vein: 10-15 cm.
> Subclavian vein: 10 cm.
> Femoral vein: 35-45 cm.

7. Run a continuous monitoring strip to accurately record pressures as the PA catheter is advanced.

8. Advance the inflated balloon, while monitoring pressures and wave forms. Watch for ventricular ectopy during insertion. Advance the catheter through the right ventricle into the main pulmonary artery until the catheter enters a distal branch of the pulmonary artery and is stopped by impaction (as evidenced by a pulmonary wedge pressure wave form).

9. Do not advance catheter with balloon deflated, and do not withdraw the catheter with the balloon inflated. After placement, obtain a chest X-ray to insure that the tip of catheter is no farther than 3-5 cm from mid-line, and no pneumothorax is present.

NORMAL PULMONARY ARTERY CATHETER VALUES

Right atrial pressure	1-7 mm Hg
RVP systolic	15-25 mm Hg
RVP diastolic	8-15 mm Hg
Pulmonary artery pressure	
PAP systolic	15-25 mm Hg
PAP diastolic	8-15 mm Hg
PAP mean	10-20 mm Hg
PCWP	6-12 mm Hg
Cardiac output	3.5-5.5 L/min
Cardiac index	2.0-3.2 L/min/m²
Systemic Vascular Resistance	800-1200 dyne/sec/cm²

INFECTION

General Considerations: In septic patients, manage airway, breathing, and circulation appropriately. Administer fluids, pressors, and ventilatory support as indicated.

Labs: Blood cultures x 2; 4 blood cultures if possible endocarditis. Urine for U/A, C&S.

Culture: Central lines, drainage catheters, pleural effusions, ascites, spinal fluid, wounds/sinuses, abscesses, cysts, sputum, heparin locks, IV lines, urine, wounds.

Consider Antibiotics: After cultures are drawn.

Post-op fever 5 W's: Water - UTI; Wind-pneumonia; Wound-inspect wound carefully for infection; Walking - pulmonary embolus; Wonder drugs-drug fevers.

Antibiotic Strategies: Check culture results if available; nosocomial infections require broad spectrum antibiotics until culture results. Consider source of infection before choosing an antibiotic.

Consider:HIV status, underlying disorders, immunosuppression, renal failure, endocarditis or meningitis.

HYPERTENSION

Assessment: Recheck blood pressure; determine if medication was recently discontinued; check current medications.

Symptoms of end-organ damage: Neurologic (lethargy, headache), Cardiac (angina), or Renal (hematuria).

Treatment:

A. Manage underlying pain, agitation, delirium tremens, hypoxemia. Use caution in the setting of recent neurologic events, the brain may need elevated pressure.

B. Attempt to lower the diastolic pressure to 100 within an hour, further reduction should be gradual.

C. Add or increase antihypertensive or nitrate therapy.

HYPOTENSION

Support: Airway, Breathing, Circulation, and start oxygen. Establish monitors for blood pressure, pulse respirations. Call Code if patient is unstable.

Establish IV and Consider Fluid bolus: 250 cc NS IV over 1 hour. Make sure pressors are being administered through working IV line. Stop nitroglycerin drips, remove nitroglycerine paste.

Labs: EKG, portable CXR; ABG; glucose, electrolytes, calcium, Mg, CBC.

Correct Hypoglycemia: D5W. Reverse narcosis (naloxone 2 mg).

CARDIOLOGY

By Kirk Voelker, MD

MYOCARDIAL INFARCTION & UNSTABLE ANGINA

Labs: SMA 12, magnesium; fasting lipids (LDL, HDL triglycerides). Cardiac enzymes: CPK, CPK-MB q6h x 24h & qd until peak. LDH & isoenzymes. CBC, PT/PTT, UA. ECG (with V_4R if inferior posterior involvement), repeat if chest pain or q30-60min if MI in evolution is suspected. CXR, echocardiogram.

Diet: Cardiac diet, 2 gm sodium, low fat, low cholesterol diet. No caffeine or temperature extremes. NPO if unstable.

THROMBOLYTIC THERAPY IN MYOCARDIAL INFARCTION
Inclusion Criteria:

A. Chest pain typical of acute myocardial infarction for longer than 30 min.

B. Electrocardiography: Changes consistent with acute myocardial infarction (ST-segment elevation ≥ 1 mV in two contiguous leads) or presence of left bundle-branch block pattern.

C. Presence of inferior infarction -- ST segment elevation of ≥ 2 mm in leads 2, 3 and AVF with ≥ 2 mm ST segment depression in leads V1-V4 and ST elevation of ≥ 1 mm in leads V3R, V4R (right ventricular MI).

D. Age may exceed 75 years.

E. Late initiation of treatment is appropriate (up to 24 hours after MI).

Contraindications:
Relative

Absence of ST-segment elevation

Severe hypertension

Cerebrovascular disease

Relatively recent surgery more than 2 weeks prior

Cardiopulmonary resuscitation

Absolute

Active internal bleeding

History of hemorrhagic stroke

Head trauma

Pregnancy

Surgery within 2 weeks

Recent noncompressible vascular puncture

Labs: PTT q6h. Fibrinogen q6h until normalized. Type and cross 2 units PRBC's.

Precautions: No IM injections, no arterial punctures; watch IV sites for bleeding

Thrombolytics:

A. Streptokinase or Anistreplase (APSAC):

Lower incidence of intracerebral hemorrhage than tPA in patients ≥75 years of age.

1. Aspirin 325 mg chew and swallow now and qd **AND**
   Heparin 5000 U IV push **AND**
   Diphenhydramine 50 mg IV push **AND**
   Methylprednisolone 250 mg IV push.
2. Streptokinase-1.5 million IU of streptokinase in 100 mL NS IV over 60 min **OR**
   Anistreplase-30 units IV over 2-5min.
3. Heparin 10 U/kg/h IV infusion immediately after administration of streptokinase or anistreplase and maintain PTT 1.5-2 times control.
4. PTT, fibrinogen now **AND** q6h x 24h. No IM or arterial punctures, watch IV for bleeding.

B. Recombinant Tissue Plasminogen Activator (tPA):

Most beneficial for myocardial infarction with less than 4 hours from onset of chest pain. Higher incidence of intracerebral hemorrhage than streptokinase in patients ≥75 years of age.

1. Aspirin, 325 mg chew and swallow now & qd. Heparin 5000 U IV bolus
2. Reconstitute 100 mg tPA (50 mg tPA/vial): tPA 15 mg IVP over 2 min, followed by 0.75 mg/Kg (max 50 mg) IV infusion over 30 min, followed by 0.5 mg/Kg (max 35 mg) IV infusion over 60 min (total dose ≤ 100 mg).
3. Start heparin 15 U/kg/h IV infusion after tPA, & adjust to PTT of 1.5-2 times control.
4. PTT & fibrinogen now & q6h x 24h. No IM or arterial punctures, watch IV for bleeding.

Oxygen, Morphine, Nitroglycerine:

-Oxygen 2-4 L/min by NC

-Nitroglycerine Drip 15 µg IV bolus, then 5 µg/min infusion (50 mg in 250-500 mL D5W, 100-200 µg/mL). Titrate upward in 5-10 µg/min steps, up to 200-300 µg/min; maintain MAP >80 or systolic >90; titrate to control symptoms; keep increase in heart rate to less than 20% of baseline rate **OR**

-Nitroglycerine SL, 0.4 mg (0.15-0.6 mg) SL q5min until pain free (up to 3 tabs)

-Isosorbide dinitrate (Isordil) 10-60 mg PO q6-8h [5,10,20, 30,40 mg]; **OR**

-Nitroglycerine ointment (2%) ½-2 inch q4-8h **OR**

-Nitroglycerine Patch (Transderm-Nitro) 0.1-0.6 mg/h qd. Place patch on in AM and off before bedtime to prevent NTG tolerance [0.1, 0.2,0.3, 0.4, 0.6 mg/h patches].

-Morphine sulfate 2-4 mg slow IV q5-10 min until pain free.

Beta Blockers:
-Metoprolol (Lopressor) 5 mg IV q2-5 min x 3 doses; then 25 mg PO q6h x 48h, then 100 mg PO q12h, titrate to HR < 60, may give 2 mg IV q2h prn pulse > 70, hold if systolic <90 **OR**

-Esmolol hydrochloride (Brevibloc) 500 µg/kg IV over 1 min, then 50 µg/kg/min IV infusion titrated to HR of <60 (max of 300 µg/kg/min) **OR**

-Propranolol 0.1 mg/kg IV divided in 3 doses q5min; followed in 1h by 20-40 mg PO q6-8h (160-240 mg/d), titrate to HR <60 **OR**

-Atenolol (Tenormin) 5-10 mg IV, then 50-100 mg PO qd, titrate to HR <60 (max 200 mg/d.

-**Relative Contraindications to beta-Blockers:** Brady arrhythmias, second-third degree heart block, hypotension, bronchospastic lung disease, concurrent administration of calcium channel blockers.

Heparin and Aspirin:
-Heparin 5000 U (100 U/kg) IV bolus followed by 1000 U/hr (15 U/kg); adjust to PTT 1.5-2 times control.

-Aspirin 325 mg PO qAM, first dose chewable now.

Lidocaine:
-Lidocaine (treatment of frequent PVC's or V tach) 75-100 mg (1 mg/kg) IV over 5 min, then 40 mg (0.5 mg/kg) IV over 5 min q8-10 min prn until total of 4 mg/kg, then infuse 1.4-3.5 mg/min (20-50 µg/kg/min; 2 gm in 500 mL of D5W)

Evaluate for Thrombolytic Therapy, see page 31.

Symptomatic Medications:
-Ranitidine (Zantac) 50 mg IV q8h or 150 mg PO bid.

-Acetaminophen (Tylenol) 325-650 mg PO q4-6h prn headache.

-Lorazepam (Ativan) 1-2 mg PO tid or qid prn anxiety **OR**

-Diphenhydramine (Benadryl) 25-50 mg PO qhs prn sleep.

-Docusate (Colace) 100-250 mg PO bid.

-Dimenhydrinate (Dramamine) 25-50 mg IV over 2-5 min q4-6h or 50 mg PO q4-6h prn nausea **OR**

-Promethazine (Phenergan) 10 mg IV q4h prn nausea.

Note: If still symptomatic, obtain cardiology consult for angioplasty, bypass graft, or balloon pump.

PHARMACOLOGY OF UNSTABLE ANGINA

		Benefits		
	Reduce	Prevent	Reduce	
Drug	**Mortality**	**AMI**	**Angina**	**Disadvantages**
Aspirin	+++	+++	-------	Bleeding
Heparin	-------	+++	++	Bleeding, thrombocytopenia
Nitrates	-------	+	+++	Tolerance, hypotension
Beta-Blockers	-------	+	+++	Bronchoconstriction, AV block reduced contractility
Calcium antagonists	-------	-------	+++	Hypotension, AV block, reduced contractility, tachycardia
Lytic Therapy	++	-------	+	Bleeding

AMI = acute myocardial infarction; AV = atrioventricular

CONGESTIVE HEART FAILURE AND CARDIOGENIC SHOCK

Management of Congestive Heart Failure:

1. **Reduce Preload:** Diuresis, nitroglycerine IV, morphine IV.
2. **Reduce Afterload:** ACE inhibitors, nitroglycerine IV, nitroprusside.
3. **Increase Contractility with Inotropic Agents**: Dobutamine, milrinone,
4. **Increase myocardial O_2 Supply:** Supplemental Oxygen, mechanical ventilation, positive end expiratory pressure.
5. **Rule out Precipitating Causes of CHF:** Drugs, aortic stenosis, papillary muscle dysfunction, chordae tendineae rupture, dissecting aneurysm with aortic insufficiency
6. **Diagnostic Measures:** Swan-Ganz Catheter, Echocardiogram, ECG with V_4R, CXR, ECG

7. **Labs:** SMA 7 & 12, CBC, cardiac enzymes, ABG, iron studies. Repeat SMA 7 & 12 in AM. Digoxin level. UA. Consider thyroid function tests.

Management of Left Ventricular Diastolic Failure:

Diet: 0.5-2 gm salt cardiac diet. Fluid intake of 1-1.5 L/d.

IV Fluids: Hep-lock with flush q shift. Foley to closed drainage.

Oxygen: 2-4 L/min by NC.

Diuretics:
-Furosemide 40-80 mg IV push, double the dose if inadequate response within 30-60 minutes; or 20-80 mg PO qAM [20,40,80 mg] **OR**
-Toresemide (Demadex) 20-40 mg IV push, double the dose if no response within 30-60 minutes; or 5-20 mg PO qd; max 200 mg/day IV or PO [5, 10, 20, 100 mg]. The dose of toresemide is equal to ½ of furosemide. Torsemide has greater oral absorption and is more expensive than furosemide **OR**
-Bumetanide (Bumex) 0.5-1 mg IV q2-3h until response; then 0.5-1.0 mg IV q8-24h (max 10 mg/d); or 0.5-2.0 mg PO qAM **OR**
-Metolazone (Zaroxolyn) 2.5-10 mg PO qd, max 20 mg/d; 30 min before loop diuretic [2.5,5,10 mg].

Digoxin:
-Digoxin Loading dose (previously undigitalized) 0.25-0.5 mg IV, followed by 0.25 mg IV q6h until a total dose of 0.75-1.0 mg (8-12 mcg/kg lean body weight; 6-10 mcg/kg in renal failure).
-Digoxin Maintenance-0.125-0.5 mg PO or IV qd [0.125,0.25, 0.5 mg].

Inotropics and Pressors:
-Dobutamine 2.5-10 µg/kg/min, max of 14 µg/kg/min (500 mg in 250 mL D5W, 2 µg/mL) titrate to CO >4, CI >2 **AND/OR**
-Milrinone (Primacor) 50 mcg/Kg IV over 10 min, followed by 0.375-0.75 (average 0.5) mcg/Kg/min IV infusion (40 mg in 200 mLs NS (QS), conc=0.2 mg/mL).

Nitrates and Nitroprusside:
-Nitroglycerine 10 µg/min IV (50 mg in 250-500 mL D5W); titrated to MAP 70 systolic > 90, max 300 µg/min **OR**
-Isosorbide dinitrate (Isordil) 10-40 mg PO qid.
-Nitroprusside sodium 0.1-10 µg/kg/min IV, increase by 0.1-0.2 µg/kg/min; (50 mg in 250-500 mL D5W) titrate to CI >2-4 & CO >4. Should not be used for extended periods because thiocyanate and cyanide levels increase.

ACE-Inhibitors:
-Lisinopril (Zestril, Prinivil) 5-40 mg PO qd [5,10,20,40 mg].
-Benazepril (Lotensin) 10-40 mg PO qd, max 80 mg/d [5,10,20,40 mg].
-Fosinopril (Monopril) 10-40 mg PO qd, max 80 mg/d [10,20 mg].
-Quinapril (Accupril) Initially 5-10 mg PO qd, then 20-80 mg PO qd in 1 to 2 divided doses [5,10,20,40 mg].
-Ramipril (Altace) 2.5-10 mg PO qd, max 20 mg/d [1.25,2.5,5,10 mg].
-Losartan (Cozaar) 25-50 mg PO qd-bid, max 100 mg/day [25, 50 mg]. Does not cause couth or angioedema.
-Losartan/HCTZ (Hyzaar) one tab PO qd-bid [50/12.5 mg].
-Captopril (Capoten) 6.25-50 mg PO q8h [12.5, 25,50,100 mg].
-Enalapril (Vasotec) 1.25-5 mg slow IV push q6h or 2.5-20 mg PO bid [5,10,20 mg].

Potassium and Other Agents:
-Morphine sulfate 5-10 mg IV q2-4h or 1-4 mg IV q5min prn.
-KCl (Micro-K) 20-60 mEq PO qd.
-Magnesium Chloride (Slow-Mag) 2-4 tabs/d PO in divided doses [64 mg].

Low Dose Beta-blockers (experimental):
-Metoprolol (Lopressor) 5 mg PO qd-bid. Titrate as tolerated to 10 mg PO qd-bid [low-dosage formulations are not commercially available].

Management of Right Ventricular Infarct and RV Failure:
Give volume challenges (250 cc NS, 25 g Albumin), Dobutamine.

Symptomatic Medications:
-Docusate sodium 100-200 mg PO qhs.
-Ranitidine (Zantac) 50 mg IV q8h or 150 mg PO bid.

CONGESTIVE HEART FAILURE MANAGEMENT ALGORITHM

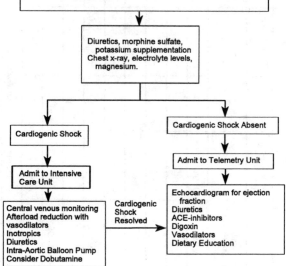

Dyspnea on exertion, paroxysmal nocturnal dyspnea, fatigue, weakness, lower extremity edema, jugular venous distension, third heart sound, rales.

Diuretics, morphine sulfate, potassium supplementation Chest x-ray, electrolyte levels, magnesium.

Cardiogenic Shock

Cardiogenic Shock Absent

Admit to Intensive Care Unit

Admit to Telemetry Unit

Central venous monitoring
Afterload reduction with vasodilators
Inotropics
Diuretics
Intra-Aortic Balloon Pump
Consider Dobutamine

Cardiogenic Shock Resolved

Echocardiogram for ejection fraction
Diuretics
ACE-inhibitors
Digoxin
Vasodilators
Dietary Education

INOTROPIC/VASOACTIVE AGENTS

Medication	Dose	Adrenergic Receptor[1]	Inotropic	Chronotropic	Vasoconstrictor	Vasodilator
Milrinone (Primacor)	50 mcg/kg IV over 10 min, followed by 0.375-0.75 mcg/kg/min IV infusion (40 mg in 200 mL NS, conc = 0.2 mg/mL)		+++	0	0	0
Dobutamine	5-15 mcg/kg/min 200 mg/250 cc D5W	B1 B2	+++	0	-	++[3]
Dopamine[4]	low dose: 1-3 mcg/kg/min	DA	0	0	0	??
	Mid dose: 3-10 mcg/kg/min	B1 B2	+++	++	0	0
	High dose: 10-20 mcg/kg/min	a B1	+++	++	+++	0
Isoproterenol	0.5-1 mcg/kg/min 1 mg/250 cc D5W	B1 B2	+++	++++	0	++
Norepinephrine	0.5-30 mcg/kg/min 4 mg/250 cc D5W	B1 a	+++	+++	++++	0
Phenylephrine	40-100 mcg/min	a	0	0	++++	0
Epinephrine	0.005-0.2 mcg/kg/min 1 mg/250 cc D5W	a B1 B2	+++	+++	++	0
	>0.2 mcg/kg/min	a B1	++++	++++	++++	0

[1]a=alpha; B₁=Beta-1; B₂=Beta-2; DA=Dopaminergic. [2]Catecholamines should not be mixed with alkaline solution
[3]May cause hypotension at doses below 15 mcg/kg/min. [4]May enhance hypoxic pulmonary vasoconstriction and increase PA pressures
[5]vasoconstriction of renal arteries only. +=mild effect; ++++=strongest effect; 0=negligible effect

CLINICAL APPROACH TO SHOCK

SHOCK   (low blood pressure, unresponsive patient)
YES ↓

ARRHYTHMIA ---> YES ---> | See Advance Cardiac life Support
NO ↓
   ↓

JVD -----> NO ---->   Volume loss due to Hemorrhage, Third Spacing,
      ↓   Sepsis, Drugs, CNS/Spinal Injury Anaphylaxis,
YES ↓   Anaphylactoid, Adrenal Insufficiency

**FLUID FILLED
LUNGS** --->   NO --->   Right Heart Failure, Right ventricular,
                          Myocardial infarction, Pulmonary embolism,
      ↓   tension Pneumothorax, PEEP, Cardiac
YES ↓   Tamponade, Superior vena cava Syndrome,
                          Right arterial Myxoma, Right Prosthetic Valve
                          Dysfunction

MURMUR ---> YES --->   Aortic insufficiency, Mitral regurgitation,
                           Papillary Muscle Dysfunction, Chordae
                           Rupture, Left Arterial Myxoma, Left Prosthetic
                           Valve Dysfunction,

NO ↓   Ventricular septal defect, aortic insufficiency
                           or stenosis, idiopathic hypertropic septal
                           stenosis

S3, S4, Rub ---> YES --->   MI/Ischemia, Cardiomyopathy
Pulsus   Myocarditis, Volume Overload
Paradoxus   Drugs, Cardiac Tamponade, Pulmonary
                                 Embolism, Constrictive Pericarditis

ATRIAL FIBRILLATION & ATRIAL FLUTTER

Labs: CBC, SMA 7 & 12; serial CPK's, MB fraction, LDH, UA, PT/PTT, TSH, T4. CXR, ECG. Echocardiogram (chamber size).

Treatment:

1. **Cardioversion:** (if patient unstable, onset <12 months, or unresponsive to drugs):

    If patient stable, start quinidine or procainamide 2-3 days prior & have patient anticoagulated (3 weeks if chronic A fib; anticoagulation not required if onset <3 days) & NPO x 6h, digoxin level ≤2.4, normal serum potassium.

2. **Sedation Prior to Cardioversion:**

    Midazolam (Versed) 2-5 mg IV or thiopental sodium (Pentothal) 2 mg/kg IVP.

3. **Synchronized Cardioversion:**

    Atrial Fibrillation.............100 J.
    Atrial Flutter..................25-50 J.

Rate Control:

-Esmolol (Brevibloc) 500 mcg/kg IV over 1 min loading dose, then 50 mg per min. If ineffective, reload and increase maintenance dosage by 25-50 mcg/kg/min to max of 300 mcg/kg/min **OR**

-Propranolol 1-5 mg (0.15 mg/kg) given IV in 1 mg aliquots min then 40-80 mg PO tid-qid. **OR**

-Metoprolol (Lopressor) 5-15 mg IV loading dose, then 25-100 mg/day PO.

-Atenolol (Tenormin) 5-10 mg IV loading dose, then 25-100 mg/day PO **OR**

-Digoxin 0.5 mg IV, then 0.25 mg IV q4h x 2-6 doses as needed until ventricular rate 60-90 bpm at rest or until 15-20 mcg/kg given; then 0.125-0.375 mg PO or IV qd **OR**

-Verapamil (Isoptin) 2.5-10 mg IV over 2-3 min (may give calcium gluconate 1 gm IV over 3-6 min prior to verapamil to counteract hypotension); then 40-120 mg PO q8h or verapamil SR 120-240 mg PO qd **OR**

-Diltiazem (Cardizem) 0.25 mg/kg IV over 2 min, then 5-15 mg/h IV infusion (100 mg in 250 mLs D5W (QS); conc 0.4 mg/mL).

Pharmacologic Conversion (after rate control and anticoagulation if >3 days duration):

-Quinidine gluconate (Quinaglute) 15 mg/kg in 150 mL D5W IV over 4-6h loading, followed by 0.8 mg/kg/h infusion (reduce dose by 25% if CHF) **OR** Quinidine sulfate 400 mg PO q 2-4h x 2 doses loading, followed by quinidine gluconate 324 mg PO q8h **OR** quinidine gluconate 330 mg PO q2-4h x 2 doses, then 330 mg IM or PO q8h **OR**

-Procainamide IV loading dose of 1000 mg (15 mg/kg) at 20 mg/min IV; then 2-6 mg/min IV maintenance; or PO loading dose: 750-1000 mg; then 250-1000 mg PO q6h (50 mg/kg/d in 4-6 divided doses) **OR**

-Amiodarone (Cordarone) 400 mg PO q8h loading dose x 10-14 days, then 200-400 mg PO qd **OR**

-Propafenone (Rythmol) 150-300 mg PO q8h, max 1200 mg/d **OR**

-Sotalol (Betapace) 80-160 mg PO bid.

Anticoagulation of Patients with Chronic Atrial Fibrillation::

-Heparin (see page 56) maintain PTT 1.5 times control **AND**

-Warfarin (Coumadin) (see page 56),maintain PT at 1.2-1.5 x control; INR 2.00-3.00.

Symptomatic Medications:

-Lorazepam (Ativan) 2 mg PO tid prn anxiety.

WOLF-PARKINSON-WHITE SYNDROME

Labs: CBC, SMA 7 & 12, ABG, UA. CXR, ECG.

Treatment:

-Attempt vagal maneuvers before drug treatment. Consider cardioversion with 50 J (see page 40) if indicated. Carotid message is contraindicated if bruit present.

-Adenosine (Adenocard) 6 mg rapid IV over 1-2 sec, followed by saline flush, may repeat 12 mg IV after 2-3 min, up to max of 30 mg total; theophylline blocks adenosine receptors **OR**

-Propafenone (Rythmol) 150-300 mg PO q8h, max 1200 mg/d **OR**

-Quinidine gluconate 15 mg/kg in 150 mL D5W over 4-6h loading, followed by 0.8 mg/kg/h infusion (reduce dose by 25% if heart failure) **OR** Quinidine sulfate 400 mg PO q 2-4h x 2 doses loading, followed by quinidine gluconate 330 mg IM or PO q8h **OR** quinidine gluconate 330 mg IM or PO q2-4h x 2 doses, then 330 mg IM or PO q8h.

-Procainamide IV loading dose 20 mg/min IV until max total of 1 gm (15 mg/kg); then 2-6 mg/min IV infusion maintenance; or PO loading dose, 750-1000 mg; then 0.5-1.0 gm PO q4-6h (50 mg/kg/d in 6-8 doses)

VENTRICULAR ARRHYTHMIAS

1. Ventricular Fibrillation & Tachycardia:

-**If unstable (see ACLS protocol page 6)**, defibrillate with unsynchronized 200 J, then 300 J.

-Oxygen 100% by mask.

-Lidocaine loading dose 50-100 mg IV, then 2-4 mg/min IV **OR**

-Procainamide loading dose 10-15 mg/kg at 20 mg/min IV or 100 mg IV q5min, then 1-6 mg/min IV maintenance **OR**

-Bretylium loading dose 5-10 mg/kg over 5-10 min, then 2-4 mg/min IV.

-Also see "other antiarrhythmics" below.

2. TORSADES DE POINTES:

-Correct underlying cause & consider discontinuing drugs that cause Torsades de pointes (quinidine, procainamide, disopyramide, moricizine, bepridil, lidocaine, amiodarone, phenothiazines, tricyclic and tetracyclic antidepressants, terfenadine, vasopressin, imidazoles, pentamidine, amantadine); correct hypokalemia and hypomagnesemia.

-Magnesium sulfate (drug of choice) 1-4 gm in IV bolus over 5-15 min or infuse 3-20 mg/min for 7-48h until QT interval <0.5 sec.

-Isoproterenol (Isuprel)(may worsen ischemia) 2-20 µg/min (2 mg in 500 mL D5W, 4 µg/mL) **OR**

-Phenytoin (Dilantin) 100-300 mg IV given in 50 mg aliquots q5min.

-Consider ventricular pacing & cardioversion.

3. Other Antiarrhythmics:

Class I:

-Moricizine (Ethmozine) 200-300 mg PO q8h, max 900 mg/d.

Class Ia:

-Quinidine sulfate 200-600 mg PO q4-6h (max 2.4 gm/d) or gluconate 324-648 mg PO q8-12h **OR**

-Procainamide PO loading dose of 750-1000 mg (15 mg/kg) in 2-3 divided doses, then 250-1000 mg PO q4-6h or 1 gm IV load given as 100 mg IV q5min or 20 mg/min until arrhythmia suppressed, then 2-6 mg/min IV infusion **OR**

-Disopyramide 100-300 mg PO q6-8h.

Class Ib:

-Lidocaine (50-100 mg IV, then 2-4 mg/min IV) **OR**

-Mexiletine (Mexitil) 100-200 mg PO q8h, max 1200 mg/d **OR**

-Tocainide (Tonocard) loading 400-600 mg PO, then 400-600 mg PO q8-12h; max 1800 mg/d **OR**

-Phenytoin, loading dose 100-300 mg IV given as 50 mg in NS over 10 min IV q5min, then 100 mg IV q5min prn.

Class Ic:

-Flecainide (Tambocor) 50-100 mg PO q12h, max 400 mg/d.

-Propafenone (Rythmol) 150-300 mg PO q8h, max 1200 mg/d.

Class II:

-Propranolol 1-3 mg IV in NS (max 0.15 mg/kg) or 20-80 mg PO q6h (80-160 mg/d) **OR**

-Esmolol loading dose 500 µg/kg over 1 min, then 50 µg/kg/min IV infusion, titrate to max 300 mcg/kg/min **OR**

-Atenolol 50-100 mg/d PO **OR**

-Nadolol 40-100 mg PO qd-bid **OR**

-Metoprolol 50-100 mg PO bid-tid **OR**

-Timolol 5-10 mg PO bid.

Class III:

-Amiodarone (Cordarone) PO loading 400-1200 mg/d in divided doses x 5-14 days, then 200-400 mg PO qd (5-10 mg/kg) **OR**
-Sotalol (Betapace) 40-80 mg PO bid, max 320 mg/d in 2 divided doses.
-Bretylium 5-10 mg/kg IV over 5-10 min, then maintenance of 1-4 mg/min IV or repeat boluses 5-10 mg/kg IV q6-8h; infusion of 1-4 mg/min IV.

Labs: SMA 12, Mg, calcium, CBC, cardiac enzymes, LFT's, ABG, drug levels, thyroid function test. UA. CXR, ECG, signal averaged ECG, electrophysiologic study.

PERICARDITIS

Labs: CBC, SMA 12, albumin, UA. Viral serologies: Coxsackie A & B, echo, measles, mumps, influenza, ASO titer, hepatitis surface antigen, ANA, rheumatoid factor, anti-myocardial antibody, PPD with candida, mumps. Cardiac enzymes q8h x 4, ESR, complement CH-50, thyroid panel, PT/PTT, blood C&S X 2.

Pericardiocentesis: Gram stain, C&S, Thayer-Martin, cell count & differential, cytology, glucose, protein, LDH, amylase, triglyceride, AFB, fungal, specific gravity, pH, LE prep, rheumatoid factor. Obtain cardiology/cardiothoracic surgical consult when possible for pericardiocenteses. ECG, echocardiogram, CXR PA & LAT.

Treatment:

Nonpurulent Pericarditis:
-Aspirin 650 mg PO q4-6h (2-3 gm/d) **OR**
-Indomethacin 25-75 mg PO tid **OR**
-Ibuprofen 400 mg PO tid or qid
-Morphine 2-4 mg IV q5-10 min; narcotics should be used cautiously if possible tamponade or constriction-may cause hypotension **OR**
-Meperidine 50-100 mg IV q3-4h prn pain and Promethazine (Phenergan) 25-75 mg IV q4h.
-Prednisone 40-60 mg PO qd. Evaluate for infectious causes prior to considering initiating steroids.

Purulent Pericarditis:
-Nafcillin or Oxacillin 2 gm IV q4h **AND EITHER**
-Gentamicin or Tobramycin 100-120 mg IV (1.5-2 mg/kg); then 80 mg (1.0-1.5 mg/kg) IV q8h (adjust in renal failure) **OR**
-Ceftizoxime 1-2 gm IV q8h.
-Vancomycin 1 gm IV q12h may be used in place of nafcillin or oxacillin.

HYPERTENSIVE EMERGENCY

Labs CBC, SMA 7, UA with micro. Thyroid panel, urine metanephrines, serum renin. Urine drug screen. CXR, ECG, renal Doppler & scan.

Treatment of Specific Hypertensive Syndromes:

A. **Aortic Dissection:** Lower systolic blood pressure to between 100 and 110 mm Hg with nitroprusside unless myocardial or cerebral ischemia. Consult a cardiologist and thoracic surgeon.

B. **Unstable Angina:**
   1. Initiate oxygen, nitroglycerin drip, aspirin, and intravenous beta blockers.
   2. Nitroprusside is contraindicated in myocardial infarction because of coronary steal phenomenon. Heparin should not be used until after the diastolic blood pressure is less than 110 mm Hg.

C. **Acute Myocardial Infarction:**
   1. Very high blood pressure may be reduced by treatment of pain and anxiety with nitrates, morphine, and a benzodiazepine; pressure >110 mmHg.
   2. Treat with oxygen, IV nitroglycerin, IV metoprolol or atenolol, aspirin. Thrombolytic therapy should not be started until the blood pressure has been lowered >110 mmHg.
   3. Nitroprusside is contraindicated in myocardial infarction because of coronary steal phenomenon.

D. **Hypertension with Pulmonary Edema:** Treatment systolic heart failure with IV furosemide, morphine, nitrates, digoxin, oxygen, nitroprusside; oral ACE-inhibitor therapy.

E. **Renal Syndromes:** If the patient is not volume-depleted, initiate parenteral therapy with a loop diuretic. Avoid nitroprusside in patients with impaired renal function because of the risk of thiocyanate toxicity.

F. **Hyperadrenergic States:**
   1. **Differential Diagnosis:**
      a. Pheochromocytoma, sympathomimetic drug toxicity (amphetamine, pheniramine, phenylpropanolamine, ephedrine, phenylephrine, cocaine).
      b. **MAO-inhibitor** interactions occur with tyramine-containing foods, sympathomimetic agents, methyldopa, dopamine and levodopa.
      c. Withdrawal from clonidine (Catapres), or methyldopa (Aldomet) and cocaine use.
   2. Labetalol or nitroprusside are the best choices because of simplicity of use; however, phentolamine (2-5 mg IV) is a more specific for alpha-receptor blockade.

3. Cocaine toxicity responds well to IV labetalol because it reduces excess catecholamine activity induced by sympathomimetic drug use, and may also reduce the risk of cardiac arrhythmia.

4. Before beginning labetalol for any hyperadrenergic state, consider whether pheochromocytoma is a possibility. Urine for metanephrines must be obtained before initiating labetalol therapy because the drug will affect urinary metabolites.

5. If the BP elevation can be traced to withdrawal from clonidine HCL (Catapres), the best option is to reinstitute the drug.

Hypertensive Drug Therapy:

-**Nitroprusside sodium** 0.25-10 µg/kg/min IV (50 mg in 250 mL of D5W), titrate to desired BP. Avoid acute fall in BP.

-**Nitroglycerine** 5-100 µg/min IV, titrated to chest pain or desired BP, up to 300 µg/min (50 mg in 250-500 mL D5W).

-**Labetalol** (Trandate) 20 mg IV bolus (0.25 mg/kg), then 20-80 mg boluses IV q10-15 min titrated to desired BP Infusion of 0.5-2 mg/min; then 100-400 mg PO bid.

-**Clonidine** (Catapres), initial 0.1-0.2 mg PO followed by 0.05-0.1 mg per hour until DBP <115 (Max total dose of 0.8 mg); then 0.1-2.4 mg/d in divided doses bid-tid, max 2.4 mg/d.

-**Propranolol** (Inderal) 1-10 mg load, then 3 mg/h IV, then 80-640 mg/d PO in divided doses.

-**Nifedipine** (Procardia) 5-20 mg PO repeat prn; then 10-30 mg PO q8-6h, max dose of 120 mg/d **OR** extended release (Procardia XL) 30-60 mg PO qd, max 120 mg [30,60,90 mg].

-**Verapamil** (Calan) 5 mcg/kg/min IV infusion, then 40-80 mg PO tid, max 360 mg/d [40,80,120 mg] or Sustained release 120-240 mg PO qd, max 240 mg PO bid [240 mg].

-**Phentolamine** [pheochromocytoma (alpha blockade)], 5-10 mg IV, repeated as needed up to 20 mg.

-**Trimethaphan camsylate** (Arfonad)(dissecting aneurysm) 2-4 mg/min IV infusion (500 mg in 500 mL D5W).

TEMPORARY PACEMAKERS

Temporary Pacemakers: Placed acutely for life threatening conduction blocks and bradycardia, and are sometimes placed prophylactically during the acute phase of MI.

Transvenous Pacemakers: Inserted into the right heart via the subclavian, femoral vein, or jugular veins. The generator is attached to the leads.

External Pacemakers-Place one paddle posteriorly between the scapulae, and the other on the sternum. Temporary measure until a transvenous pacer can be inserted.

Indications:

Prophylactic: New right bundle branch block (RBBB) with left heart block (LHB), alternating bundle branch block (BBB), Mobitz type II, complete heart block (CHB).

Therapeutic: Symptomatic bradycardia unresponsive to medical therapy. Heart rate < 50 with symptoms. Sequential pacing of atria and ventricles when hemodynamically compromised by AV dissociation.

Management of Transvenous Pacer Problems:

-If the patient is unstable, place the external pacer paddles on and turn output up until capture occurs.

-If the pacer does not capture, turn the output to maximum voltage. If that fails, try turning the sensitivity up (lower threshold voltage). Change batteries or change units.

-Order daily potable CXR to rule out pneumothorax and check lead placement.

-Record daily threshold measurements

PERMANENT PACEMAKERS

General Considerations: Leads placed transvenously either in the right
ventricle, right atrium, or both. Leads are attached to a pulse generator;
sutured below the skin.

Five Position Pacemaker Code:

Clamber Paced	Chamber Sensed	Response to Sensing	Programmable functions	Anti-tachy-functions
Ventricle	Ventricle	Triggers	Programmable	Programmable
Atrium	Atrium	Inhibits	Multiprogrammable	Shock
Double	Double	Double: T or I	Communicates	Double: P and S
O-none	O-none	O-none	Rate modulation	

Most pacemakers are VVI or DDD.

Indications:

Complete heart block (regardless of symptoms).

Mobitz II if symptomatic

BBB with or without symptoms (depending on patterns)

Sick Sinus Syndrome if symptomatic. or if beta blocker or Calcium blocker
therapy is planned

Carotid sinus hypersensitivity if symptomatic.

Post pacemaker implantation:

Immediate and daily CXR should be ordered to rule out pneumothorax and
evaluate lead position. Check wound condition daily.

REFERENCES

Selvester RHS. The Twelve Lead ECG and Initiation of Thrombolytic Therapy for Acute
Myocardial Infarction. J of Electrocardiography 1993 Vol 26 (supl) 114-120.

Gonzalez ER. Pharmacologic controversies in CPR. Annals of Emergency Medicine.
[JC:4z7] 22(2 Pt 2):317-23. 1993 Feb.

Anonymous. Guidelines for cardiopulmonary resuscitation and emergency cardiac care.
Emergency Cardiac Care Committee and Subcommittees, American Heart
Association... Part III. Adult advanced. cardiac life support JAMA [JC:kfr] 268(16)
:2199-241, 1992 Oct 28

Ornato JP Use of adrenergic agonists during CPR in adults. Medical College of Virginia,
Richmond. Annals of Emergency Medicine. [JC:4z7] 22(2 Pt 2):411-6, 1993 Feb.

The GUSTO Investigators: An international randomized trial comparing four thrombolytic
strategies for acute myocardial infarction. N Engl J Med 1993; 329: 673-682.

Chatterjee K. Complications of acute myocardial infarction. Current Problems In Cardiology
[JC:dvd]18(11:1-79, 1993 Jan.

Murdock CJ. Klein GJ. Yee R. Leitch JW. Management of the patient with the
Wolff-Parkinson-White syndrome. Cardiology. [JC:coil] 77(3) :151-65, 1990.

Pritchett EL. Management of atrial fibrillation. New England Journal of Medicine. [JC:now]
326(19):1264-71, 1992 May 7.

Reeder GS, Gersh BJ. modern management of acute myocardial infarction. Current
Problems in Cardiology [JC:dvd] 18(2):81-155, 1993 Feb.

Ram CV. Management of hypertensive emergencies: changing therapeutic options.
American Heart Journal. [JC:3bw] 122(1 Pt 2):356-63, 1991 Jul.

PULMONOLOGY

By Theodore Shankel, MD

AIRWAY MANAGEMENT AND INTUBATION

<u>Oral Tracheal Intubation:</u>
ETT Size (<u>interior diameter</u>):

Women 7.0-9.0 mm

Men 8.0 -10.0 mm.

1. **Prepare functioning suction** apparatus set-up and ready. Have bag and mask apparatus set-up with 100% oxygen; and ensure that patient can be adequately bagged and suction apparatus is available.

2. **If sedation and/or paralysis is required,** consider rapid sequence induction as follows:

   -Fentanyl (Sublimaze) 50 mcg increments IV (1 mcg/kg) **with:**

   -Midazolam hydrochloride (Versed) 1 mg IV q2-3 min, max 0.1-0.15 mg/kg **followed by:**

   -Succinylcholine (Anectine) 0.6-1.0 mg/kg. Succinylcholine may cause hyperkalemia (see contraindications in package insert).

   Note: These drugs may cause vomiting; therefore, apply cricoid cartilage pressure during intubation (Sellick maneuver).

3. **Position patient's head** in "sniffing" position with head flexed at neck and extended. If necessary elevate head with a small pillow.

4. **Bag patient** with bag mask apparatus and hyper-oxygenate with 100% oxygen.

5. **Hold Endoscope** handle with left hand, and use right hand to open patient's mouth. Insert along right side of mouth to the base of tongue, and push tongue to the left. Advance to the vallecula (superior to epiglottis, if using curved blade) and lift anteriorly, being careful not to exert pressure on the teeth. If using a straight blade, place beneath the epiglottis and lift anteriorly, avoiding the teeth.

6. **Place endotracheal tube (ETT)** into right corner of mouth and pass through the vocal cords; stop just after the cuff disappears behind vocal cords. If unsuccessful after 30 seconds, stop and resume bag and mask ventilation before reattempting. If necessary, use stilette to maintain the shape of the ETT (a hockey stick shape may be helpful); remove stilette after intubation.

7. **Inflate cuff with syringe** keeping cuff pressure $\leq$ 20 cm H_2O and attach the tube to an Ambu bag or ventilator. Confirm bilateral, equal expansion of chest and equal bilateral breath sounds. Auscultate abdomen to confirm that the ETT is not in the esophagus. If there is any question about proper ETT location, repeat laryngoscopy with tube in place to be sure it is

endotracheal; remove tube immediately if there is any doubt about proper location. Secure the tube with tape and note centimeter mark at the mouth. Suction the oropharynx and trachea.

8. **Confirm placement** with a chest X-ray (tip of ETT should be between the carina and thoracic inlet, or level with the top of the aortic notch).

Nasotracheal Intubation:

Nasotracheal intubation may be preferred method if prolonged intubation is anticipated (increased patient comfort). Intubation will be facilitated if patient is awake and spontaneously breathing. There is an increased incidence of sinusitis with nasotrachael intubation.

1. **Spray nasal passage with vasoconstrictor:** cocaine 4%, 4 cc **OR** Phenylephrine 0.25% (Neo-Synephrine) 2.3 cc unless contraindicated. If sedation is required before nasotracheal intubation, administer fentanyl (Sublimaze) 1 mcg/kg with midazolam hydrochloride (Versed) 0.05-0.1 mg/kg.

   Lubricate nasal airway with lidocaine ointment.

   Tube Size:
   Women   7.0 mm tube
   Men 8.0, 9.0 mm tube

2. **Place the nasotracheal tube** into the nasal passage and guide it into nasopharynx along a U-shaped path. Monitor breath sounds by listening and feeling the end of tube. As the tube enters the oropharynx, gradually guide the tube downward. If the sounds stop, withdraw the tube 1-2 cm until breath sounds are heard again. Reposition the tube, and, if necessary, extend the head and advance. If difficulty is encountered, perform direct laryngoscopy and insert under direct visualization, or use Magill forceps.

3. **Successful intubation occurs** when the tube passes through the cords; a cough may occur and breath sounds will reach maximum intensity if the tube is correctly positioned. Confirm correct placement by checking for bilateral breath sounds and expansion of chest.

4. **Confirm placement with chest x-ray.**

RESPIRATORY FAILURE AND VENTILATOR MANAGEMENT

1. **Indications for Ventilatory Support:** Respirations > 35, VC < 15 mL/kg, negative inspiratory force $\leq$ -25, pO2 < 60 on 50% O_2, pH < 7.2, $pCO_2 \geq$ 55, severe, progressive, symptomatic hypercapnia and/or hypoxia.

2. **Intubation:** Prepare suction apparatus, laryngoscope, endotracheal tube ($\geq$ No. 8 if possible); clear airway and place oral airway, hyperventilate with bag and mask attached to high flow oxygen.
   Midazolam (Versed) 1-2 mg IV boluses until sedated.
   Intubate, inflate cuff, ventilate with bag, auscultate chest, suction.

3. **Initial Orders:** FiO_2 = 100%, PEEP = 3-5 cm H_2O, assist control 8-14 breaths/min, tidal volume = 800 mL (10-15 mL/kg ideal body weight), set rate so that minute ventilation (VE) is approximately 10 L/min. Alternatively, use intermittent mandatory ventilation mode with tidal volume and rate to achieve near-total ventilatory support. Consider pressure support in addition to IMV at 5-15 cm H_2O.

4. **If Decreased Minute Ventilation:** Evaluate patient and rule out complications (endotracheal tube malposition, cuff leak, secretions, bronchospasms, pneumothorax, worsening pulmonary disease, sedative drugs, pulmonary infection). Readjust ventilator rate to maintain mechanically assisted minute ventilation of 10 L/min. If peak AWP is > 45 cm H_2O at outset, consider decreasing tidal volume to 7-8 mL/kg (with increase in rate if necessary), or decreasing ventilator flow rate.

5. **ABG** in 30 min, CXR for tube placement, measure cuff pressure q8h (maintain $\leq$ 20 mm Hg), pulse oximeter, arterial line, and/or monitor end tidal CO_2. Maintain oxygen saturation > 90-95%.

6. **If Arterial Saturation $\geq$ 94% & pO$_2$ > 100,** reduce FIO_2 (each 1% decrease in FIO_2 reduces pO$_2$ by up to 7 mm Hg); once FIO_2 < 60% may reduce PEEP by increments of 2 cm H_2O until PEEP = 3-5 cm H_2O. Maintain O_2 saturation of $\geq$ 90% (pO$_2$ > 60).

7. **If arterial saturation < 90% & pO$_2$ < 60,** increase FIO_2 up to 60-100%, then consider increasing PEEP by increments of 3-5 cm H_2O (if PEEP >10 consider PA catheter). Add additional PEEP until oxygenation is adequate with an FIO_2 of < 60%. PEEP may be detrimental in patients with severe obstructive lung disease, increased intracranial pressure, and left ventricular dysfunction. PEEP decreases cardiac output resulting in decreased hepatic metabolism of theophylline, lidocaine, and other agents that undergo extensive hepatic drug clearance.

8. **If pH is Excessively Low,** (pH < 7.33 due to respiratory acidosis/hypercapnia) increase rate and/or tidal volume. Keep peak airway pressure < 40-50 cm H_2O if possible. For severe lung impairment consider alkalinization and permissive hypercarbia.

9. **If pH is High,** (> 7.48 due to respiratory alkalosis/hypocapnia) reduce rate and/or tidal volume to lessen hyperventilation. If patient is breathing rapidly above ventilator rate, it may be necessary to change to IMV from AC, or sedate patient.

10. **If Patient is "Fighting" Ventilator,** despite appropriate sensitivity, flow rate settings and tidal volume, consider IMV or SIMV mode, or add sedation with or without paralysis (exclude complications or other causes of agitation). Never use paralytic agents without concurrent amnesia and/or sedation.

11. **Sedation** (if pH >7.55):

   -Diazepam (Valium) 2-5 mg slow IV q2h prn agitation, max dose 20-30 mg **OR**

   -Lorazepam (Ativan) 1-2 mg IV q1-2h prn sedation **OR**

   -Midazolam (Versed) 1-2 mg IV boluses until sedated **OR**

   -Thiopental 50 mg IV test dose, then 2-4 mg/kg IV **OR**

   -Methohexital 50-120 mg IV **OR**

   -Pentobarbital drip 5 mg/kg/h IV for 1-2h, then 0.5-1.0 mg/kg/h IV infusion; maintain sedative pentobarbital level of 3-5 mg/L.

   -Morphine Sulfate 2-5 mg IV q5min, max dose 20-30 mg **OR** 0.03-0.05 mg/kg/h IV infusion (50-100 mg in 500 mL D5W) titrated **OR**

   -Propofol (Diprivan): 50 mcg/kg bolus over 5 min, then 5-50 mcg/kg/min.

12. **Paralysis** (with simultaneous sedation and/or amnesia)

   -Succinylcholine (Anectine) 0.6-1.0 mg/kg; very short acting, $T\frac{1}{2}$ 3.5 min **OR**

   -Atracurium (Tracrium) 0.5 mg/kg IV, then 0.3-0.6 mg/kg/h infusion; short acting, $T\frac{1}{2}$ 20 min; due to histamine releasing properties, may cause bronchospasm and/or hypotension **OR**

   -Vecuronium (Norcuron) 0.1 mg/kg IV, then 0.06 mg/kg/h IV infusion or q1h prn; intermediate acting, $T\frac{1}{2}$ 60 min; hepatic/renal elimination **OR**

   -Pancuronium bromide (Pavulon) 0.08 mg/kg IV, then 0.03 mg/kg/h infusion or q1h IV prn; long acting, $T\frac{1}{2}$ 75 min; renal elimination; may cause tachycardia and/or hypertension.

   Note: Monitor level of paralysis with a peripheral nerve stimulator using the "train-of-four (TOF) mode. Adjust neuromuscular blocker dosage to achieve TOF 90-95%; if patient on inverse ratio ventilation, maintain TOF at 100%.

13. **Loss of Tidal Volume**: If a difference between the tidal volume setting and the delivered volume occurs, check for a leak in the ventilator or inspiratory line. Check for a poor seal between the endotracheal tube cuff or malposition of the cuff in the subglottic area. If a chest tube is present, check for air leak.

14. **Daily weaning parameters** if indicated.

INVERSE RATIO VENTILATION

1. **Possible Indications:** Some combination of pAO_2 <60 mm Hg, FIO_2 > 0.6, peak airway pressure > 45 cm H_2O, or PEEP > 15 cm H_2O. Requires heavy sedation and muscle relaxation.

2. **Set oxygen concentration** (FIO_2) at 1.0; inspiratory pressure at ½ to 2/3 the peak airway pressure on standard ventilation; set the inspiration: expiration ratio at 1:1; set rate at ≤ 15 breaths/min. Maintain tidal volume by adjusting inspiratory pressures. Monitor auto-PEEP level.

3. **Monitor** PaO_2, oxygen saturation (by pulse oximetry), $PaCO_2$, end tidal PCO_2, PEEP, mean airway pressure, heart rate, blood pressure, SVQ, and cardiac output.

4. **If SaO_2 remains** < 0.9, consider increasing I:E ratio (2:1, 3:1), but generally attempt to keep I:E ratio ≤ 2:1. If SaO_2 remains <0.9, increase PEEP or return to conventional mode. If $PaCO_2$ is excessively high, evaluate tracings to determine appropriate management. If hypotension develops, rule out tension pneumothorax, administer intravascular volume or pressor agents, decrease I:E ratio or return to conventional ventilation mode.

VENTILATOR WEANING

Ventilator Weaning Parameters to be checked Before Attempting to Wean Patient (general guidelines, adjustments must be made for individuals based on clinical condition):

1. Patient alert and rested.
2. PAO_2 >70 mm Hg on FiO_2 <50%.
3. $PaCO_2$ <50 mm Hg; pH >7.25.
4. Negative Inspiratory Force (NIF) more negative than -20 cm H_2O.
5. Vital Capacity >10-15 mL/kg (800-1000 mL).
6. Minute Ventilation (VE) <10 L/min; respirations <24 breaths per min (at steady state).
7. Maximum voluntary minute ventilation double that of resting minute ventilation.
8. PEEP ≤ 5 cm H_2O.
9. Tidal volume 5-8 mL/kg.
10. RR/V_T < 105.
11. No chest wall or cardiovascular instability, or excessive secretions.
12. Ability to guard airway must be assured.

Terminate Weaning Trial if any of the Following Occurs:

1. PAO_2 falls below 55 mm Hg.

2. Acute hypercapnia.
3. Deterioration of vital signs or clinical status (arrhythmia).
4. Patient requests being placed back on ventilator (if clinically appropriate).

Rapid T-tube Weaning Method for Short-term (<7 days) Ventilator Patients without Chronic Obstructive Pulmonary Disease:

1. Obtain baseline respiratory rate, pulse, blood pressure and arterial blood gases or oximetry. Discontinue sedation, have patient sit in bed or chair, and well rested. Provide bronchodilators, theophylline, and suctioning if indicated.
2. Attach endotracheal tube to a T-tube with an inspired oxygen concentration 10% greater than previous level; T-tube flow should exceed peak inspiratory flow.
3. After initial 5 minute interval of spontaneous ventilation, resume mechanical ventilation and draw an arterial blood gas sample (unless gas-exchange is being continuously monitored).
4. If the 5 minute blood gas is acceptable, a 15 minute interval may be attempted. If the 15 minute interval blood gas is adequate, a 30 minute interval may be attempted. After each interval the patient is placed back on the ventilator for an equal amount of time.
5. If the 30 minute interval blood gas is acceptable and the patient is without dyspnea, a 2-hour period may be attempted; and if blood gases are acceptable, extubation may be considered.

T-tube Weaning Method for Prolonged Ventilator Patients or Chronic Obstructive Pulmonary Disease:

1. Continue the above weaning trial after the 5 minute and 15 minute intervals; if successful, follow by a 30 minute, 1 hour, 2 hour, 4 hour, 8 hour and 16 hour interval; evaluate arterial blood gas after each interval during the day. If patient deteriorates at any time, return to last successful interval.
2. When patient is able to breathe for 24 hours with acceptable blood gases and without deterioration, extubation may be considered. With T-tube method the weaning trial is not successful unless the PAO_2 remains >55 mmHg without worsening hypercapnia.

Intermittent Mandatory Ventilation Weaning Method (IMV):

1. Obtain baseline vital signs, and arterial blood gases or pulse oximetry. Discontinue sedation; consider pressure support of 10-15 cm H_2O. Change the ventilator from assist control to intermittent mandatory ventilation mode; or if already on intermittent mandatory ventilation, decrease the rate as follows:

Patients with No Underlying Lung Disease and on Ventilator for a Brief Period ($\leq$1 Week):

1. Decrease IMV rate at 30 min intervals by 1-3 breaths per min at each step, starting at a rate of 8 breaths per minute until a rate of zero is

reached. If each step is well tolerated and arterial blood gases are adequate (pH >7.30 or 7.35), extubation may be considered when IMV rate is zero.

Patients with Chronic Obstructive Pulmonary Disease or Prolonged

Ventilator Support for ≥1 week:

1. Begin IMV at frequency 8 breaths/minute, with a tidal volume of each mandatory breath of 10 mL/kg, with an oxygen concentration 10% greater than previous rate. Monitor end tidal CO_2.

2. Blood gases should be drawn at 30 and 60 minutes after changing to a rate of 8 breaths per minute. If patient tolerates the decreased rate poorly or if arterial blood gases deteriorate, the IMV should be increased until patient's blood gases stabilize.

3. If the patient is able to tolerate a decreased IMV to 8 breaths/minute after 60 minutes, the IMV rate may be decreased to 6 breaths/min with repeat monitoring of arterial blood gases after 30 and 60 min; or monitor end tidal CO_2 and pulse oximetry.

4. If the patient remains stable, IMV may be decreased to 4 breaths/min followed by 2 breaths per minute; Repeat arterial blood gases drawn at 30 and 60 minute intervals.

5. If patient tolerates the IMV rate of zero without deterioration in vital signs or blood gases, a T-tube may be placed, and observe patient for an additional 24 hours before being extubated.

6. If deterioration occurs, increase IMV to previously stable rate until following morning, then reconsider weaning if indicated.

Pressure Support Ventilation:

1. Pressure support ventilation is initiated on an empiric basis at 5-25 cm H_2O. Set level to maintain the spontaneous tidal volume at 7-15 mL/kg.

2. Gradually decrease the level of pressure support ventilation in increments of 3-6 cm H_2O according to the ability of the patient to maintain satisfactory minute ventilation. Extubation can be considered at a pressure support ventilation level of 5 cm H_2O.

Problems Associated with Inability to Wean Patient from Ventilator:

Bronchospasms, active pulmonary infection, secretions, small endotracheal tube, weakness of respiratory muscle, low cardiac output.

NEAR DROWNING

1. **Maintain airway**, ventilation, and stabilize circulation.
2. **If History of Initial Loss of Consciousness,** alteration in cognitive function or trauma to head or neck, consider spinal cord injury until ruled out.
3. **If Symptoms of Cardiopulmonary Instability,** provide adequate oxygen by mask or intubate, and give 100% oxygen ventilation. Administer cardiac massage if necessary. Insert a nasogastric tube to remove ingested water from the stomach.
4. **Obtain Chest X-rays, Arterial Blood Gases, Electrolytes,** establish intravenous access. If continued hypoxemia on 100% oxygen by mask, consider intubation and administer 40-50% oxygen, followed by repeat arterial blood gases.
5. **Fluid Resuscitation** may be necessary with lactated Ringer's or normal saline. Inotropic support with dopamine may be necessary. Electrolyte abnormalities such as dilutional hyponatremia may occur if a large volume of fresh water is absorbed from the gastrointestinal tract. Urine output should be monitored with a Foley catheter. Diuretics should generally be avoided for treating pulmonary edema as they may worsen hypovolemia. If peripheral perfusion is poor, a plasma volume expander, such as human plasma protein fraction should be provided.
6. **If Persistent Hypoxemia <60 mm Hg despite** maximal ventilation, correct by providing positive end-expiratory pressure; initially consider 5-10 cm H_2O and adjust as needed. If metabolic acidosis with pH <7.1, administer intravenous bicarbonate 1-2 mEq/kg.
7. **Hypothermia** should be treated by drying patient; removal of wet clothing: and blankets. If core temperature is $32°$-$35°$ C, active external warming should be initiated with a heating blanket or radiant warmer. If the core temperature is <$32°$ C, active internal rewarming should be added, including heated aerosolized oxygen, heated intravenous fluids, gastric lavage, and peritoneal dialysis. Drowning victims should not be declared dead, until a core temperature of $36°$ C has been reached without recovery. Consider emergency cardiopulmonary bypass.
8. **Criteria for Hospitalization:** History of apnea or cyanosis, CPR, loss of consciousness, hypoxemia, acidosis, abnormal chest x-ray or physical exam.
9. **General Measures:** High-dose broad spectrum antibiotic therapy may be indicated if evidence of aspiration exist or for empiric treatment of suspected infection. Steroids are usually not indicated, but methylprednisolone, 30 mg/kg IV over 30 min may be used. Provide respiratory therapy with bronchodilators, and assist with coughing and deep breathing. Gastric activity should be maintained at pH >4.5 with H_2 blockers or antacids.

PULMONARY EMBOLISM

Labs: CXR PA & LAT, ECG, VQ scan, impedance plethysmography, Doppler scan of legs, venography, pulmonary angiography. CBC, INR/PTT, SMA7, ABG, cardiac enzymes, UA.

Treatment:

Pulse oximeter, guaiac stools; O_2 at 2-4 L by NC, maintaining O_2 sat >90%. Determine underlying cause of thrombotic disease.

Anticoagulation:

-Heparin IV bolus 5000-10,000 U (100 U/kg ideal body weight) then 1000-2000 U/h (20 U/kg/h if <70 years, 15 U/kg/h if $\geq$ 70 [25,000 U in 250 or 500 mL D5W (50-100 U/mL)]; adjust q4-6h to PTT 1.5-2.5 times control (45-75 sec) x 7-10 days. Draw PTT 6 hours after bolus & q4-6h until PTT 1.5-2.5 x control, then qd or q12h. Check PT at initiation of warfarin & qd.

-Warfarin (Coumadin) 5-10 mg PO qd x 2-3 days, then 2-7.5 mg PO qd based on rate of rise of INR. Maintain INR 2.0-3.0 (INR of 3.0-4.5 if recurrent pulmonary embolism). Patients should be adequately heparinized prior to starting Coumadin.

-**Anticoagulant overdose** (see page 83)

Streptokinase (indicated for hemodynamic compromise):

1. Baseline CBC, PT/PTT, fibrinogen, thrombin time, UA; acetaminophen 650 mg 1-2 tabs PO q4-6h prn; methylprednisolone 250 mg IV, diphenhydramine 50 mg IV.
2. Streptokinase, 250,000 units IV over 30 min, then 100,000 units/h for 24-72 hours, followed by heparin (see below) without IV bolus.
3. Draw PTT, thrombin time, fibrinogen, fibrin split products 4h after start of infusion, and then q4-6h. If PTT or thrombin time >5 x control, discontinue; if PTT or thrombin time <2 x control, reload with 500,000 units. If PTT <2 x control after 2nd loading dose, discontinue streptokinase, and use heparin or urokinase.
4. Discontinue infusion after 24h, PTT or thrombin time after 1h. When PTT is <2 times control, initiate **Heparin** infusion at 10 U/kg/h & gradually increase as fibrinogen is restored to maintain PTT 1.5-2.5 x control (**no loading dose**).
5. Thrombolytic therapy promotes faster resolution of thrombus but does not alter long-term outcome.

Symptomatic Medications:

-Meperidine 25-100 mg IV prn pain.
-Docusate sodium (Colace) 100-200 mg PO qhs.
-Ranitidine (Zantac) 150 mg PO bid.

-Avoid intramuscular injections.

ASTHMA

Labs: ABG, CBC, SMA7, phosphate, theophylline level. Sputum Gram stain, C&S. CXR, pulmonary function test with bronchodilators, ECG.

Treatment:

-Oxygen 2-6 L/min by NC. Keeping SaO_2 >90%. Monitor peak flow rate before and after bronchodilator treatments; monitor pulse oximeter.

Beta Agonists:

-Albuterol (Ventolin, Proventil)l nebulized, 0.2-0.5 mL (2.5 mg) in 3 mL saline initially, then q2-8h (5 mg/mL sln) **OR**

-Albuterol (Ventolin, Proventil) or Metaproterenol (Alupent) MDI up to 20 puffs over a 10-20 min treatment period, repeated every 20-30 min then 1 puff q1-10min. Patients must be continuously monitored for side effects; cardiac arrhythmias, tremor, and hypokalemia. Then 2 puffs q1-6h or powder 200 mcg/capsule inhaled qid. Beta agonists should be changed to a prn basis as soon as patient has stabilized.

-Salmeterol (Serevant) 2 puffs q12h; beneficial for prophylaxis of exercise-induced or nocturnal asthma; should not be used in acute asthma due to slow onset of action.

Corticosteroids and Ipratropium:

-Methylprednisolone (Solu-Medrol) 40-125 mg IV q6h; then 30-60 mg PO qd **OR**

-Prednisone 40-60 mg PO qAM.

-Beclomethasone (Beclovent) MDI 2-6 puffs qid, with spacer 5 min after bronchodilator, followed by gargling with water **OR**

-Triamcinolone (Azmacort) MDI 1-4 puffs tid-qid **OR**

-Flunisolide (AeroBid) MDI 2-4 puffs bid **OR**

-Budesonide MDI 200-800 mcg qid.

-Metered dose corticosteroids should be the mainstay of treatment after patient has stabilized.

-Ipratropium (Atrovent) 2-4 puffs q4-6h.

Aminophylline & Theophylline:

-Aminophylline loading dose: 5.6 mg/kg **total** body weight in 100 mL D5W IV over 20-30 min (if patient not previously on theophylline preparations). Maintenance of 0.5-0.6 mg/kg (**ideal** body weight)/h (500 mg in 250 mL D5W); reduce if elderly, heart/liver failure (0.2-0.4 mg/kg/hr); may need up to 0.8-0.9 mg/kg/h if young and/or smoker. Reduce load by 50-75% if taking theophylline (1 mg/kg of aminophylline will raise levels 2 µg/mL) **OR**

-Theophylline IV solution loading dose 4.5 mg/kg **total** body weight, then 0.4-
  0.5 mg/kg (**ideal body weight**)/hr.
-Theophylline (Theo-Dur) PO loading dose of 6 mg/kg, then maintenance of
  100-400 mg PO bid-tid (3 mg/kg q8h); 80% of total daily IV aminophylline
  in 2-3 doses.

Acute Bronchitis:
-Ampicillin 0.5-1 gm IV q6h or 250-500 mg PO qid **OR**
-Ampicillin/sulbactam (Unasyn) 1.5 gm IV q6h **OR**
-Cefuroxime (Zinacef) 750-1500 mg IVPB q8h **OR**
-Clarithromycin (Biaxin) 250-500 mg PO bid [250, 500 mg] **OR**
-Cefuroxime axetil (Ceftin) 250-500 mg PO bid [250, 500 mg]

Symptomatic Medications:
-Docusate sodium (Colace) 100-200 mg PO qhs.
-Ranitidine (Zantac) 50 mg IV q8h or 150 mg PO bid or other antacid/H_2
  blocker prophylaxis.

CHRONIC OBSTRUCTIVE PULMONARY DISEASE

Labs:
ABG, CBC, phosphate, SMA7, UA. Theophylline level stat & after 12-24h of
  infusion & 24-48h after PO. Sputum Gram stain & C&S. CXR, PFT's with
  bronchodilators, ECG, PPD with controls. Peak flow rate pre & post
  bronchodilators, pulse oximeter.

Treatment:
-O_2 1-2 L/min by NC or 24-35% by Venturi mask, keep O_2 saturation 90-
  91%. Use oxygen cautiously if chronic hypercapnia.

Acute Beta-Agonist Therapy:
-Nebulized Albuterol (Ventolin, Proventil) or 0.2-0.5 mL in 3 mL (2.5 mg) of
  saline [with unit dose of ipratropium (Atrovent)] initially, then q2-8h (5
  mg/mL sln) **OR**
-Albuterol (Ventolin, Proventil) MDI 2-8 puffs then 2 puffs; then 2 puffs q4-
  6h; add ipratropium (Atrovent), 2-4 puffs q4-6h **OR**
-Taper beta agonists to as needed as soon as patient has stabilized.

Aminophylline & Theophylline:
-Aminophylline loading dose-5.6 mg/kg **total** body weight over 20-30 min (if
  not on theophylline preparations); then 0.5-0.6 mg/kg (**ideal** body
  weight)/hr (500 mg in 250 mL of D5W); reduce if elderly, heart or liver
  disease (0.2-0.4 mg/kg/hr). Reduce loading by 50-75% if already taking
  theophylline (1 mg/kg of aminophylline will raise level by 2 µg/mL) **OR**
-Theophylline IV solution loading dose 4.5 mg/kg **total** body weight, then 0.4-
  0.5 mg/kg (**ideal** body weight)/hr.

-Theophylline long acting (Theo-Dur) PO loading dose of 6 mg/kg, then maintenance of 100-400 mg PO bid-tid (3 mg/kg q8h); 80% of daily IV aminophylline in 2-3 doses.

Corticosteroids & Anticholinergics:

-Methylprednisolone (Solu-Medrol) 40-60 mg IV q6h or 30-60 mg PO qd **OR**

-Prednisone 40-60 mg PO qd, taper to minimum dose.

-Triamcinolone (Azmacort) MDI 2-4 puffs qid **OR**

-Beclomethasone (Beclovent) MDI 2-6 puffs qid, with spacer, 5 min after bronchodilator, followed by gargling with water **OR**

-Atropine 1-2 mg in 1 cc NS by nebulizer q4h **OR**

-Ipratropium Bromide (Atrovent) MDI 2 puffs tid-qid.

Acute Bronchitis:

-Ampicillin 1 gm IV q6h or 250-500 mg PO qid **OR**

-Trimethoprim/Sulfamethoxazole (Septra DS) 160/800 mg PO bid or 160/800 mg DS IV q8-12h (6-10 mg TMP/kg/d)(10-15 mL of IV sln in 100 cc D5W tid; 16 mg/mL) **OR**

-Ampicillin/sulbactam (Unasyn) 1.5 gm IV q6h **OR**

-Cefuroxime 0.75-1.5 gm IV q8h.

Symptomatic Medications:

-Docusate sodium (Colace) 100-200 mg PO qhs.

-Ranitidine (Zantac) 50 mg IV q8h or 150 mg PO bid.

HEMOPTYSIS

General Measures:

A. Consider otolaryngology consult to rule out upper airway etiology. Obtain immediate thoracic surgical consult for massive hemoptysis.

B. If hemoptysis is moderate, place patient on bedrest with sedation, adequate cough suppression, avoidance of excessive chest manipulation, and consider antibiotics.

C. Keep patient in lateral decubitus, bleeding side down if >200 mL/day volume hemoptysis.

D. Quantify all sputum & blood, suction prn. Endotracheal tube (8 mm) ready, O_2 at 100% by mask, pulse oximeter. Have double lumen endotracheal tube available for use.

Treatment:

1. Transfuse packed red blood cells as needed.

2. Codeine 15-30 mg PO q4-6h (cough suppression may be contraindicated in patients with massive hemoptysis). **OR**
   -Hydrocodone 5 mg PO q4-6h.

3. Consider empiric antibiotics if any suggestion that bronchitis or infection may be contributing to hemoptysis.
4. Correct any coagulation disorders (except if pulmonary embolism is the cause).

Labs: Type & cross 4-6 U PRBC. ABG, CBC, platelets, SMA7 & 12, ESR, Anti-glomerular basement membrane antibody, rheumatoid factor, complement, cryoglobulins, antineutrophil cytoplasmic antibody (ANCA). Sputum Gram stain, C&S, AFB, parasites & fungal, & cytology x 3, sputum pH. UA, PT/PTT. CXR PA, LAT, ECG, VQ scan, contrast CT, technetium scan, bronchoscopy. PPD & controls.

ACUTE PULMONARY EDEMA

General Measures:
-Keep patient sitting or in semi-Fowler position. I&O, O_2 at 100% by mask, pulse oximeter.
-Consider intubation and positive pressure ventilation (PEEP)

Treatment:
Diuretics:
-Furosemide 10-80 mg IV bolus over 1-2 minutes q30 min (double dose prn), max total of 1 gm/d **OR**
-Toresemide (Demadex) 20-40 mg IV push, double the dose if no response within 30-60 minutes; or 5-20 mg PO qd; max 200 mg/day IV or PO [5, 10, 20, 100 mg]. The dose of toresemide is equal to ½ of furosemide. Torsemide has greater oral absorption and is more expensive than furosemide **OR**
-Bumetanide (Bumex) 0.5-1.0 mg IV q2-3h until response occurs, then 0.5-1.0 mg IV q8-24h (max 10 mg/d); or 0.5-2.0 mg PO qAM.
-Metolazone (Zaroxolyn) 2.5-10 mg PO qd, max 20 mg/d; 30 min before loop diuretic [2.5,5,10 mg].

Inotropics:
-Digoxin Loading dose 0.25-0.5 mg IV, followed by 0.25 mg IV q6h until a total dose of 0.75-1.0 mg (if not already on digoxin) (8-12 mcg/kg lean body weight; 6-10 mcg/kg in renal failure).
-Digoxin Maintenance-0.125-0.5 mg PO or IV qd (adjust based on serum levels); digoxin loading is not exclusive of beta inotropic agents.

Inotropic Agents:
-Dopamine 1-20 µg/kg/min IV (200 mg in 250 cc D5W, 800 µg/mL), titrate to systolic > 90, CI >2-4, CO >4.
-Dobutamine 2.5-10 µg/kg/min, max of 14 µg/kg/min (500 mg in 250 mL D5W, 2 µg/mL).

-Milrinone (Primacor) 50 mcg/kg IV over 10 min, followed by 0.375-0.75
  mcg/kg/min IV infusion (40 mg in 200 mLs NS (QS), conc = 0.2 mg/mL)
-Watch for signs of worsening ischemia or tachycardia.

Bronchodilators:

-Albuterol or Metaproterenol 0.2-0.3 mL in 3 mL of saline nebulized q30-60
  min initially, then q4-8h.

Afterload & Preload Reducers:

-Nitroglycerine 25 µg IV bolus, followed by 5-10 µg/min (100 mg in 250 mL,
  400 µg/mL). Titrate up to 100-200 µg/min in 10-20 µg/min steps.
-Nitroprusside sodium 0.1-10 µg/kg/min IV, increase by 0.1-0.5 mcg/kg/min
  (50 mg in 250-500 mL D5W) titrate to CI >2-4 & CO >4. Monitor cyanide
  and thiocyanate levels if prolonged use.
-Enalapril (Vasotec) 1.25-5 mg slow IV push q6h or 2.5-20 mg PO bid
  [5,10,20 mg].

Other Agents:

-Morphine sulfate 1-4 mg IV q5min prn initially, then q2-4h prn.
-KCl 20-40 mEq PO qAM.

Labs:

CBC, SMA 7 & 12, albumin, drug levels. ABG. Cardiac enzymes now & q8h
x 3, blood C&S x 2; sputum Gram stain, C&S, colloid osmotic pressure,
ESR. CXR, ECG.

PLEURAL EFFUSION

Labs: CBC, ABG, SMA 12, protein, albumin, amylase, rheumatoid factor, ANA,
ESR, PT/PTT, UA. Fungal serologies. CXR PA & LAT repeat after
thoracentesis, bilateral decubitus, ECG, ultrasound; PPD & candida, mumps.

Pleural fluid:

Tube 1-LDH, protein, amylase, triglyceride, glucose, (10 mL).

Tube 2-Gram stain, C&S, AFB, fungal C&S, wet mount (20-60 mL,
  heparinized).

Tube 3-Cell count and differential (5-10 mL, EDTA).

Tube 4-Sudan stain, LE prep, antigen tests for S pneumoniae, H influenza
  (25-50 mL, heparinized).

Syringe-pH (2 mL collected anaerobically, heparinized on ice)

Bag or Bottle-cytology.

Evaluation of Pleural Fluid:

Pleural Fluid Parameter	Transudate	Exudate
Pleural fluid protein/serum protein	< 0.5	> 0.5
Pleural fluid LDH	< 200	> 200
Pleural fluid LDH/serum LDH	< 0.6	> 0.6

Differential Diagnosis Includes:

Transudate: Congestive heart failure, cirrhosis.

Exudate: Empyema, viral pleuritis, tuberculosis, neoplasm, uremia, drug reaction, asbestosis, sarcoidosis, collagen disease (lupus, rheumatoid disease), pancreatitis, subphrenic abscess.

REFERENCES

Marino PL. The ICU book. Philadelphia Lea and Febiger, 1991; 329-351.

Balestrieri FJ. Analgesics. In: Chernow B ed. Essentials of critical care pharmacology. 2nd ed. Baltimore: Williams and Wilkins, 1989; 449-464.

Kaur S; Heard SO; Welch GW. In: Rippe JM; Irwin RS; Alpert JS; Fink MP. Intensive care medicine. 2nd ed. Boston: Little, Brown and Company, 1991; 10-11.

Ranieri VM; Eissa NT; Corbeil C; Chasse M; Braidy J; Matar N; Milic Emili J. Effects of positive end expiratory pressure on alveolar recruitment and gas exchange in patients with the adult respiratory distress syndrome. American Review of Respiratory Disease. 1991 Sep. 144(3 Pt 1):544-51.

Lichtwarck AM; Nielsen JB; Sjostrand UH; Edgren EL. An experimental randomized study of five different ventilatory modes in a piglet model of severe respiratory distress. Intensive Care Medicine, 1992, 18(6):330-47.

Marcy TW; Marini JJ. Inverse ratio ventilation in ARDS. Rationale and implementation. Chest, 1991 Aug, 100(2):404-504.

Yang KL; Tobin MJ. A prospective study of indexes predicting the outcome of trials of weaning from mechanical ventilation. New England Journal of Medicine, 1991 May 23, 324(21):1445-50.

MacIntyre NR. Clinically available new strategies for mechanical ventilatory support. Chest, 1993 Aug, 104(2):500-5.

Levin DL; Morriss FC; Toro LO; Drink LW; Turner CR. Drowning and near drowning. Pediatric Clinics of North America, 1993 Apr, 40(2):321-30.

Matzdorff AC; Green D. Deep vein thrombosis and pulmonary embolism: prevention, diagnosis, and treatment. Geriatrics, 1992 Aug, 47(8):48-52, 55-7, 62-3.

McFadden ER Jr; Gilbert IA. Asthma. New England Journal of Medicine. 1992 Dec 31, 327(27):1920-37.

Petty TL. Definitions in chronic obstructive pulmonary disease. Clinics in Chest Medicine. 1990 Sep, 11(3):303-73.

Clausen JL. In: Bordow RA; Moser KM. Manual of clinical problems in pulmonary medicine eds. 3rd ed. Boston: Little, Brown and Company, 1991; 67-71.

TRAUMA

By Fady G. Kadifa, M.D.

HEAD TRAUMA

I. **Acute Management of Head Trauma:**

A. Take a complete history, including the mechanism of injury, past medical history, drug intake.

B. Maintain airway, breathing and circulation; control cervical spine. Make initial assessment of the patient.

C. Assume a cervical spine injury in any patient with multisystem trauma especially injury involving the area above the clavicles. A normal neurologic examination does not rule out a cervical spine injury.

D. Perform a mini neurologic examination as soon as possible and repeat frequently. Check for lateralizing extremity weakness and pupillary function.

E. **Assess Level of consciousness (Glasgow Coma Scale):**

≤ 8	Severe head injury
9-12	Moderate head injury
13-15	Minor head injury

F. Examine skull for clinically detectable depressed, skull fracture; Battle's sign (blood in the ear canal or ecchymosis over mastoid process), Raccoon's eye (periorbital ecchymosis), rhinorrhea.

II. **Secondary Management of Head Trauma:**

A. **If Glasgow Coma Scale (GCS) is ≥ 9, pupils are equal, no lateralizing deficits, no open head injuries, the patient is neurologically intact with no loss of consciousness, or loss of consciousness less than 15 minutes and has no major underlying medical problems:** Usually represents a minor concussion. The patient may be eligible for discharge to home with instructions, provided adequate support available and access for return is possible.

B. **If GCS is ≥ 9, pupils are equal, no lateralizing deficits, no open head injuries, but neurologically not intact:** Usually represents a contusion or a small mass lesion (subdural or epidural hematomas). Requires admission for observation, neurosurgical consultation, and elective CT of head.

C. **If GCS is ≥ 9, pupils are equal, but the patient has an open head injury:** Usually caused by a basilar skull fracture or a penetrating injury. Patient needs admission with an urgent neurosurgical consultation and CT of head.

D. **If GCS is ≥ 9 but the patient has either unequal pupils or any lateralizing deficit:** Indicates possible mass effect (large subdural or epidural hematomas or an intracerebral bleed). The patient requires admission to the ICU after an urgent neurosurgical consultation and Head CT.

E. **If GCS is ≤ 8 with or without unequal pupils, lateralizing deficits or Open Head Injury:** Most likely a large intracerebral mass or a diffuse axonal injury. This patient requires ICU admission after obtaining a STAT CT of head and a STAT neurosurgical consultation. Emergency intubation is usually required for airway control with or without hyperventilation. Intubation should be done either nasally (if the patient is spontaneously breathing and no suspicion of basal skull fracture), or orotracheally with on-line-traction to keep the cervical spine straight at all times (do not hyperextend neck); consider tracheostomy.

III. Supportive Care of Head Trauma Patients:

A. Large bore intravenous access. Consider central venous pressure monitoring (CVP line or pulmonary artery catheter); consider insertion of arterial line.

B. Aggressively resuscitate shock, and search for the underlying causes (head injuries do not usually cause shock except in terminal stages).

C. Draw blood for CBC, PT, PTT, Chem 18; type and cross matching; toxicology screen, serum osmolarity.

D. Intravenous resuscitation solutions should be isotonic (lactated Ringers or normal saline). Except for shock management, consider restricting fluid intake to maintenance levels, or as indicated by hemodynamic monitoring.

E. Supply high flow oxygen. Keep patient NPO.

F. Give stress ulcer prophylaxis in the form of H_2-blockers (ranitidine, cimetidine), or sucralfate.

G. Avoid excitement, agitation, administration of sedative-hypnotics, narcotics, or neuromuscular blockers.

H. Control hyperthermia aggressively with cooling blankets.

I. Clean and repair open head wounds. Give Tetanus prophylaxis with 0.5 cc tetanus toxoid IM, with or without tetanus Ig 250 IU. IM as indicated.

IV. Management of Head Trauma Complications:

A. Elevated intracranial pressure should be treated with diuretic therapy (furosemide), hyperosmolar therapy (mannitol 1 mg/Kg IVP), or hyperventilation (maintain PCO_2 30-35 mm Hg).

B. If seizures occur, treat with lorazepam 4-8 mg IVP repeatedly until seizures are controlled, followed by phenytoin 20 mg/kg IV loading at a rate of 50 mg/min.

C. If altered mental status, give 50 mLs of 50% dextrose, thiamine 100 mg, and naloxone (Narcan) 0.4-2.0 mg, intravenously.

ABDOMINAL TRAUMA

I. **History and Physical Examination:**

    A. Up to 20% of patients with an acute hemoperitoneum will have a benign abdominal examination when first examined in the emergency department. Therefore, a negative physical examination does not preclude a significant intra-abdominal injury. Assume abdominal visceral injury in any patient sustaining a significant decelerating injury or penetrating torso wound.

    B. Take a complete detailed history, including the time of the injury; mechanism and estimated speed of impact; type of restraining devices, vehicle damage, type of weapons used; and amount of blood at the scene.

    C. The physical examination should be very thorough, with complete inspection of the whole undressed patient. An abdominal auscultation, palpation, and digital rectal examination should be performed (to assess prostate in men); vaginal examination should be completed for women

II. **General Management of Abdominal Trauma:**

    A. Control and manage airway (with cervical spine control), breathing and circulation must take priority. Constantly reevaluate patient. Deliver high flow oxygen.

    B. Insert 2 large-bore intravenous lines or preferably a central venous catheter.

    C. Send blood for CBC with differential; PT, PTT; type and cross matching; chem 18, amylase, and toxicology screen; and pregnancy test for women; chest X-ray, KUB.

    D. Insert a gastric tube (examine aspirate for blood) and a Foley catheter (examine for blood). Blind insertion of a Foley catheter is contraindicated if a high riding prostate gland on rectal exam, blood around the urethral meatus, or scrotal hematoma. Place gastric tube orally (not nasally), if maxillary bone fractures or basal skull fractures.

    E. Aggressively resuscitate shock with normal saline or lactated Ringer's infused wide open. Consider unmatched O negative blood if severe stage IV shock until properly cross-matched blood products are available.

    F. Transfuse blood products as soon as available if refractory stage III or IV shock nonresponsive to fluid challenges: i.e. 2 liters of normal saline given wide open. Do not use vasoactive substances until adequate fluid resuscitation has been given.

    G. Routine empiric use of fresh frozen plasma or platelet transfusions is unwarranted and possibly dangerous, even after massive blood transfusions unless there is active bleeding that is not controllable by other measures.

    H. Control all external sites of bleeding. Give tetanus prophylaxis if needed.

III. **Blunt Abdominal Injuries:**

    A. **If acute abdomen or pneumoperitoneum are present:** Arrange for emergency exploratory laparotomy.

    B. **If abdominal examination is equivocal (lower thoracic bruising), unreliable (head injury or intoxicated patient), or impractical, or if there is evidence of unexplained hypotension or blood loss:** Diagnostic Peritoneal Lavage (DPL) should be done or obtain a CT of the abdomen.

    C. **Criteria for Positive Diagnostic Peritoneal Lavage:**

        1. Aspiration of > 5 mL of frank blood
        2. Aspiration of obvious enteral contents: Bile, feces, undigested food particles.
        3. DPL fluid exiting from a chest tube or Foley catheter.
        4. Laboratory analysis revealing: RBC's > 100,000 cells/mm^3, WBC's 500/mm^3, amylase > 175 IU.

        Note: DPL is falsely negative in 2% of cases, most commonly due to injuries to the pancreas, duodenum, small bowel, and bladder.

IV. **Gunshot Wounds to the Abdomen:**

    A. Resuscitate as above. An aggressive policy of abdominal exploration is justified.

    B. All gunshot wounds require a laparotomy (celiotomy) if there is evidence of peritoneal penetration. Tangential wounds should be surgically explored to determine peritoneal penetration.

    C. All gunshot wounds should receive broad spectrum prophylactic antibiotics.

V. **Prophylactic Antibiotic Choices:**

    -Ampicillin/sulbactam (Unasyn) 1.5-3.0 gms IV q6h Plus Gentamicin 2 mg/kg IV loading dose, then 1.5 mg/kg IV q8h **OR**

    -Cefoxitin (Mefoxin) 1-2 gms IV q6h **OR**

    -Cefotetan (Cefotan) 1-2 gms IV q12h **OR**

    -Ampicillin 1-2 gms IV q6h, Plus Gentamicin as above, Plus metronidazole 500 mg IV q6h.

VI. **Sharp Abdominal Trauma:**

    A. **Stab wounds in a stable patient with negative abdominal examination, no involvement of the peritoneum or muscle fascia on wound exploration:** Local wound care, and consider admission for 24 hours observation with serial abdominal examinations, and serial hematocrit checks.

    B. **Stab wounds in a stable patient, if wound is below the fourth intercostal space, and if fascia is penetrated on local wound exploration, then perform a DPL:** If positive, perform exploratory laparotomy, if negative, consider admission for 24 hours observation.

C. **Stab wounds with acute abdomen, or shock, or GI or GU bleeding, or evisceration of the internal organs:** Perform exploratory laparotomy.

CHEST TRAUMA

General Principles:
A. Take a thorough history including the mechanism of injury, past medical history, drug intake.
B. Airway management with concomitant cervical spine control, breathing and circulatory control and management must take priority.
C. Assess of the whole patient after stabilization.
D. **Surgical Classification of Chest Injuries:**
   1. **Immediately Life-threatening Injures:** Massive hemothorax, tension pneumothorax, open pneumothorax, airway obstruction, flail chest, cardiac tamponade.
   2. **Potentially Life-threatening Injuries:** Myocardial contusion, esophageal rupture, tracheobronchial disruption, traumatic diaphragmatic hernia, pulmonary contusion, aortic disruption.

PNEUMOTHORAX

I. **Management of Pneumothorax:**
A. **Small Primary Spontaneous Pneumothorax (<10-15%): (not associated with any known underlying pulmonary diseases). If the patient is Not Dyspneic:**
   1. Observe for 4-8 hours and repeat a chest X-ray.
   2. If the pneumothorax does not increase in size and the patient remains asymptomatic, consider discharge home with instructions to rest and curtail all strenuous activities. Return if increase in dyspnea or recurrence of chest pain.
B. **Secondary Spontaneous Pneumothorax (associated with known underlying pulmonary pathology, most commonly emphysema) or Primary Spontaneous Pneumothorax >15%, or if patient is symptomatic:**
   1. Give high flow oxygen. Perform Needle Aspiration of the pneumothorax using a 16 gauge needle with an internal polyethylene

catheter; insert in the anterior, second intercostal space in the midclavicular line.

2. Anesthetize and prep the area before inserting needle. Attach a 60 mL syringe via a 3-way stopcock, aspirate until no more air is aspirated. If no additional air can be aspirated, and the volume of aspirated air is <4 liters: occlude the catheter and observe for 4 hours.

3. If symptoms abate and chest-x-ray does not show recurrence of the pneumothorax: the catheter can be removed, and the patient can be discharged home with instructions.

4. If the aspirated air is >4 liters and additional air is aspirated without resistance, this represents an active bronchopleural fistula with continued air leak. Admission is required for insertion of a chest tube as explained below.

C. **Traumatic Pneumothorax associated with a penetrating injury, hemothorax, mechanical ventilation, tension pneumothorax, or if pneumothorax does not resolve after needle aspiration:** Give high flow oxygen and insert a chest tube, along with aggressive hemodynamic and respiratory resuscitation as indicated. Do not delay the management of a tension pneumothorax until radiographic confirmation, insert needle thoracotomy or chest tube immediately.

II. Technique of Chest Tube Insertion:

1. Place patient in supine position, with involved side elevated 10-20 degrees; abduct arm at 90 degrees. The usual site is the fourth or fifth intercostal space, between the mid-axillary and anterior axillary line (drainage of air or free fluid). The point at which the anterior axillary fold meets the chest wall is a useful guide. Consult the chest radiograph for further guidance if time permits. Alternatively, the second or third intercostal space, in the mid-clavicular line, may be used for pneumothorax drainage alone (air only).

2. Cleanse skin with Betadine iodine solution and drape the field. Determine the intrathoracic tube distance (lateral chest wall to the apices), and mark length of tube with a clamp.

3. Infiltrate 1% lidocaine into the skin, subcutaneous tissues, intercostal muscles, periosteum, and pleura using a 25-gauge needle. Use a scalpel to make a transverse skin incision, 2 centimeters wide, located over the rib just inferior to the interspace where the tube will penetrate the chest wall.

4. Using a Kelly clamp to bluntly dissect a subcutaneous tunnel, from the skin incision extending just over the superior margin of the lower rib. Avoid the nerve, artery and vein located at the upper margin of the intercostal space.

5. Bluntly dissect over the rib and penetrate the pleura with the clamp, and open the pleura 1 centimeter.

6. With a gloved finger, explore the subcutaneous tunnel, and palpate the lung medially. Exclude possible abdominal penetration, and ensure

correct location within pleural space; use finger to remove any local pleural adhesions.

7. Use the Kelly clamp to grasp the tip of the thoracostomy tube (36 F, internal diameter 12 mm), and direct it into the pleural space in a posterior, superior direction for pneumothorax evacuation. Direct tube inferiorly for pleural fluid removal. Guide the tube into the pleural space until the last hole is inside the pleural space and not inside the subcutaneous tissue.

8. Attach the tube to a underwater seal apparatus containing sterile normal saline, and adjust to 20 cm H_2O of negative pressure, or attach to suction if leak is severe. Suture the tube to the skin of the chest wall using O silk. Apply Vaseline gauze, 4 x 4 gauze sponges, and elastic tape. Obtain a chest X-ray to verify correct placement and evaluate re-expansion of lung.

9. Consider consultation for pleurodesis sclerotherapy if clinically indicated.

TENSION PNEUMOTHORAX

I. **Signs and Symptoms:**

   A. **Clinical:** Severe hemodynamic and/or respiratory compromise; contralaterally deviated trachea; decreased or absent breath sounds and hyperresonance to percussion on the affected side; jugular venous distention, asymmetrical chest wall motion with respiration.

   B. **Radiographic:** Flattening or inversion of the ipsilateral hemidiaphragm; contralateral shifting of the mediastinum; flattening of the cardio-mediastinal contour, and spreading of the ribs on the ipsilateral side.

II. **Acute Management:**

   1. A temporary large-bore IV catheter may be inserted into the ipsilateral pleural space, at the level of the second intercostal space at the mid-clavicular line, until the chest tube is placed.

   2. A chest tube should be placed emergently.

   3. Insert 2 large-bore intravenous lines. Consider intubation, central venous pressure monitoring and arterial line.

   4. Draw blood for CBC, PT, PTT, type and cross-matching, Chem 7, Toxicology screen.

   5. Send pleural fluid for hematocrit, amylase and pH (to rule out possible esophageal rupture).

   6. **Indications for Cardiothoracic Exploration:** Penetrating chest injury, persistent air leak, severe or persistent hemodynamic instability despite

aggressive fluid resuscitation, persistent active blood loss from chest tube.

MASSIVE HEMOTHORAX

Signs and Symptoms:
A. Defined as greater than 1500 mL blood lost into the thoracic cavity; most commonly secondary to penetrating injuries.
B. Absence of breath sounds and dullness to percussion occurs on the ipsilateral side; signs and symptoms of hypovolemic shock.

Management:
1. **Restore volume deficit with crystalloid and blood transfusion.**
2. **Immediately decompress the chest cavity with a chest tube.**
3. **Place** two large-bore intravenous lines or central venous access.
4. **Insert a chest tube** as described previously, except place the site of insertion at the level of the fifth or sixth intercostal space, along the midaxillary line, ipsilateral to the hemothorax. The chest tube should not be inserted through the injury site but rather in a location away from the injury.
5. **Clean and close** penetrating wounds to decrease the likelihood of tension pneumothorax.
6. **Consider thoracotomy** based on the rate of blood loss (i.e. > 200 mL/hr for 2-3 consecutive hours) rather than the initial blood loss volume or the color of the draining blood. If the site of wound penetration is medial to the nipple anteriorly or medial to the scapula posteriorly, this represents a higher probability for injury to the myocardium and the great vessels. If the great vessels or myocardium has been injured, shock may persist despite aggressive fluid resuscitation.
7. **Provide tetanus prophylaxis** and empirical antibiotic coverage for penetrating injuries.

CARDIAC TAMPONADE

General Considerations:
A. Most commonly secondary to penetrating injuries.
B. Beck's Triad: Venous pressure elevation, drop in the arterial pressure, muffled heart sounds.
C. Other signs include: Enlarged cardiac silhouette on CXR; signs and symptoms of hypovolemic shock; electromechanical dissociation (pulseless electrical activity), decreased voltage on ECG.
D. Look for the Kussmaul's sign (rise in venous pressure with inspiration). Pulsus paradoxus or elevated venous pressure may be absent when associated with hypovolemia.

Management:
A. Pericardiocentesis is indicated if patient is unresponsive to the usual resuscitation measures for hypovolemic shock, or if high likelihood of injury to the myocardium or one of the great vessels.
B. All patients who have a positive pericardiocentesis (recovery of non-clotting blood) due to trauma, require open thoracotomy with inspection of the myocardium and the great vessels.
C. Rule out other causes of cardiac tamponade: pericarditis, penetration of central line through vena cava, atrium, or ventricle; infection.
D. Consider other causes of hemodynamic instability that may mimic the signs and symptoms of cardiac tamponade (tension pneumothorax, massive pulmonary embolism, shock secondary to massive hemothorax) especially if unresponsive to pericardiocentesis.

PERICARDIOCENTESIS

General Considerations:
A. If acute cardiac tamponade with hemodynamic instability is suspected, pneumothorax and hemothorax should be ruled out, and emergency pericardiocentesis should be performed; infusion of Ringer's lactate, crystalloid, colloid and/or blood may provide temporizing measures.

Management:
1. Protect airway, administer oxygen, and have intubation and cardiopulmonary resuscitation equipment available. If patient can be stabilized, pericardiocentesis should be performed by a specialist in the operating room or catheter lab. Intubation is very high risk in tamponade patients, and should be performed by an anesthesiologist if time permits. Use the para-xiphoid approach for pericardiocentesis in most situations.

2. Place patient in supine position with chest elevated at 30-45 degrees, then cleanse and drape peri-xiphoid area. Infiltrate lidocaine 1% with or without epinephrine (if time permits) into skin and deep tissues.

3. Attach a long, large bore (12-18 cm, 16-18 gauge), short bevel cardiac needle to a 50 cc syringe with a 3-way stop cock. Use a alligator clip to attach a V-lead of the ECG to the metal of the needle.

4. Paraxiphoid Approach: Advance the needle just below costal margin, immediately to the left and inferior to the xiphoid process. Apply suction to the syringe while advancing the needle slowly at a 45 degree horizontal angle towards the mid point of the left clavicle.

5. As the needle penetrates the pericardium, resistance will be felt, and a characteristic "popping" sensation will be noted.

6. Monitor the ECG for ST segment elevation (indicating ventricular heart muscle contact); or PR segment elevation (indicating atrial epicardial contact). After the needle comes in contact with the epicardium, withdraw the needle slightly. Ectopic ventricular beats are associated with cardiac penetration.

7. Aspirate as much blood as possible. Blood from the pericardial space usually will not clot. Blood, inadvertently, drawn from inside the ventricles or atrium usually will clot. If fluid is not obtained, redirect the needle toward the right shoulder or head.

8. Stabilize the needle by attaching a hemostat or Kelly clamp.

9. Consider emergency thoracotomy to determine the cause of hemopericardium (especially if active bleeding). If patient does not improve, consider other problems that may resemble tamponade, such as tension pneumothorax, pulmonary embolism, or shock secondary to massive hemothorax.

PULMONARY CONTUSION

General Considerations:

A. Chest x-ray reveals localized alveolar and or interstitial infiltrate, usually underlying the site of blunt injury or within the trajectory of the penetrating injury.

B. Diagnosis is usually delayed because respiratory failure develops over time rather than occurring early; severe forms may be indistinguishable from adult respiratory distress syndrome

Management:

A. Consider conservative management with close observation in a critical care unit

B. Indications for Intubation: Severe respiratory failure, preexisting chronic pulmonary disease, renal failure, abdominal injury, head trauma with secondary depressed level of consciousness..

MYOCARDIAL CONTUSION

General Considerations:
-Suspect if any blunt trauma to chest, especially if fractures or contusion of sternum or anterior ribs.
-Diagnosis may be made by ECG changes (myocardial injury, dysrhythmias, bundle branch blocks), serial enzymes, 2 D-echocardiogram (focal or regional wall motion abnormalities).

Treatment:
-Observe with supportive measures ensuring adequate oxygenation; correct of all electrolyte abnormalities; aggressively manage emerging dysrhythmias.

AORTIC RUPTURE

General Considerations:
-Tends to happen at the level of the ligamentum arteriosum; 90% mortality at the accident scene.
-Survivors usually have a contained hematoma.
-Maintain a very high index of suspicion especially in the settings of a decelerating injury.
-**Radiographic signs of Aortic Rupture:** tracheal deviation to the right; fractures of the first or second ribs; widened mediastinum; obliteration of the aortic knob; presence of a pleural cap; depression of the left main stem bronchus; obliteration of the space between the pulmonary artery and the aorta, elevation and rightward shift of the right main stem bronchus; deviation of the esophagus to the right. Frequent association with fractures of the left 1st or 2nd ribs.

Treatment:
-Obtain immediate cardiothoracic surgery consultation for thoracotomy.

TRACHEOBRONCHIAL TREE INJURY

General Considerations:
-Suspect tracheobronchial tree injury in all upper torso, penetrating or blunt (especially decelerating) injuries.

Signs and Symptoms:
-Subcutaneous emphysema; hoarseness, palpable fracture crepitus, hemoptysis.
-Check for associated injuries to the esophagus, carotid arteries, or jugular veins.
-Tension pneumothorax (especially if large air leak through chest tube).
-Abnormal breathing suggestive of airway obstruction.

Treatment:
-Maintain a high index of suspicion; secure airway and ventilation, relieve tension pneumothorax, and obtain early surgical correction of large vessel injury or esophageal disruption.

ESOPHAGEAL INJURY

General Considerations:
-Usually associated with chest penetrating injuries or severe blunt trauma to the abdomen, or instrumentation of the esophagus with nasogastric tubes or endoscopy.

Signs and Symptoms:
-After rupture, esophageal contents leak into the mediastinum followed by immediate or delayed rupture into the pleural space (usually on left), with resulting empyema.

Treatment:
1. High index of suspicion is required, look for signs of severe blows to the abdomen associated with left or sometimes right pleural effusion on chest X-ray, subcutaneous or mediastinal emphysema; shock.
2. Surgical therapy consists of primary repair if feasible, or esophageal diversion in the neck and a gastrostomy.
3. Empiric broad spectrum antibiotic therapy should be initiated as soon as possible.

FLAIL CHEST

General Considerations:

- Usually secondary to severe, blunt chest injury with multiple rib fractures (in series or bilateral), resulting in a freely moving rib segment without bony continuity with the rest of the chest wall. The segment moves in a paradoxical fashion with respect to the chest as a whole.
- Uncomplicated flail chest is usually well tolerated with no secondary hypoxia; however, major secondary dysfunctions may result from disrupted mechanical chest ventilatory function along with possible injuries to the underlying lung parenchyma (contusion and or laceration).

Treatment:

- Aggressive pulmonary toilet and close observation for any signs of respiratory insufficiency or associated major injuries.
- Treatment of complicated flail chest consists of active mechanical ventilatory support of respiration.

BURNS

I. General Burn Management:

A. Patient Stabilization:

1. Maintain airway, assess breathing and restore intravascular circulatory volume.
2. **Estimate Extent of Injury:** (Rule of 9's) 9% of total body surface area (BSA) is assigned to the head and neck, each of the upper extremities, back, both buttocks, anterior chest, abdomen, and each of the lower extremities. 1% is assigned to the perineum. First degree burns are not included in the calculation of extent of burn injury unless they represent more than 25-30 % of the BSA.

B. Assessment of Depth of Injury:

1. **First Degree Burns:** Involve the epidermis only (sunburn); blanching erythema; very painful.
2. **Second Degree Burns (Partial Thickness Burns):** Involve destruction of the epidermis with extension to various depths of the underlying dermis. Partial thickness burns are further sub-classified into superficial and deep.
3. **Third Degree Burns (Full Thickness Burns):** Involve destruction of epidermis and dermis, with extension into the subcutaneous tissue; painless; do not blanch with pressure. Third degree burns may appear pale or white or may be hard or charred.

    4. **Fourth Degree Burns**: Extend into subcutaneous tissue, muscle, fascia or bone.

II. Baseline Laboratory Evaluation of Burn Patients:
A. Arterial blood gases, CBC, Chem 20, carboxyhemoglobin level, PT and PTT, serum oncotic pressure, type and cross match, chest x-ray, ECG, UA.

III. Management of Burns:
A. Fluid Resuscitation:
1. Intravenous fluid replacement and hospitalization are required for second or third degree burns involving > 20% of the BSA. Large bore intravenous accesses (16 gauge peripheral or central lines) should be available for the fluid resuscitation.
2. Parkland Formula for calculation of the Initial Fluid Requirements: 4 mL x body weight x % second and third degree burns = total fluid deficit.

    Give 50% of the calculated deficit over the first 8 hours, then give the remaining 50% over the next 16 hours.

    Timing begins at the time of injury (not at start resuscitation).
3. Monitor vital signs closely, and observe for signs of persistent organ hypoperfusion (decreased mental status, low urine output, tachycardia, chest pain, ECG changes, peripheral vasoconstriction, persistent hyperlactemia, high anion gap metabolic acidosis.
4. If any signs of hypoperfusion are present, consider increasing fluid replacement, inotropic support, and insertion of a central venous pressure monitor, preferably a PA catheter.
5. Monitor coagulation status, serum oncotic pressure and hemoglobin/hematocrit, and replace or transfuse appropriately.

IV. Pain Control:
A. Use narcotics for pain and benzodiazepines for sedation. Titrate dosage to control pain without causing hypotension.

V. Other Considerations:
A. Tetanus prophylaxis (toxoid with or without immune globulin injections subcutaneously).
B. Place a nasogastric tube if vomiting is present, or for enteral feeding as indicated.
C. Provide appropriate peptic ulcer disease and DVT prophylaxis.

VI. Burn Care:
A. Burn wounds should be initially cleaned with copious amounts of sterile saline. Avoid vigorous scrubbing of open wounds.
B. Use sterile scissors to debride charred epithelium, remove surface debris, and excise blisters if broken; leave unbroken blisters intact.
C. Assess circumferential burns for possible fasciotomies (especially around the torso and the extremities).

D. Apply silver sulfadine cream, mafenide acetate, or silver nitrate solutions.

E. Consider consulting burn specialists, or transfer to burn centers, and consider instituting hyperbaric oxygen therapy if available

VII. Airway Burns:

A. Consider airway burns whenever burn occurs in a closed space or burns are present around the nares, mouth, or involve the face, or changes in voice, stridor, coughing up black sputum, wheezing, or signs of respiratory distress.

B. Maintain airway patency, obtain baseline arterial blood gases, chest-x-ray, carboxyhemoglobin level.

C. If stable, administer humidified 100% high-flow oxygen by mask.

D. If respiratory status is unstable, do not delay intubation and mechanical ventilation. Be ready to perform tracheostomy if necessary.

E. Fiberoptic bronchoscopy may be indicated for assessment of airway damage, airway cleaning, and to rule out foreign body aspiration.

ELECTROCUTION INJURIES

I. Acute Management of the Electrocuted Patient:

A. Admit for cardiac monitoring for the first 24-72 hours. Support airway, respiratory function, and circulation. Stabilize the neck.

B. Monitor and assess for possible undetected burns to muscle or bones. Look for burns resulting from arcing of electricity. Monitor electrolytes, chemistry panel, and urine analysis for possible signs of rhabdomyolysis (elevated CPK, aldolase, LDH, SGOT, metabolic acidosis, hypocalcemia, hyperkalemia, myoglobinuria, hemoglobinuria, renal failure).

C. Measure serial cardiac enzymes and ECG to rule out potential myocardial damage. Monitor ECG for dysrhythmias.

D. Treat thermal injuries and provide aggressive hemodynamic resuscitation with IV fluids if necessary.

E. Assess intravascular volume and urine flow with Foley catheter and maintain a urine flow of 1.0-1.5 mL/kg/h. Consider Swan-Ganz line.

F. A technetium 99 scan may be useful to exclude myocardial damage.

REFERENCES

Fulton FL: Penetrating Wounds of the Heart. Heart and Lung 1978; 7 (20: 262-268.

Jones KW: Thoracic Trauma. Surgical Clinics of North America 1980; 60-957.

Liedtke AJ, DeMuth WE: Nonpenetrating Cardiac Injuries: A collective review. American Heart Journal 1973; 86-687.

Mulder DS, Schennid H, Angood P: Thoracic Injuries, in Maull KI, Cleveland HC, Strauch GO, et al (ed): Trauma Volume 1, Chicago, Yearbook, 1986.

Committee on Trauma, American College of Surgeons: Early Care of the Injured Patient. Philadelphia, WB Sanders Co., 1982, pp 142-148.

Federle MP, Crass RA, Jeffrey B, et al: Computed Tomography in Blunt Abdominal Trauma. Archives of Surgery 1982; 645-650.

Fischer RP, Beverlin BC, Engrav LH, et al: Diagnostic Peritoneal Lavage Fourteen years and 2,586 Patients Later. American Journal of Surgery 1978; 136: 701-704.

Hill AC, Schececter WP, Trunkey DD: Abdominal Trauma and Indications for Exploratory Laparotomy, in Mattox, Moore, and Feliciano (Eds). Trauma, Rockville, Appleton-Century-Crofts, 1987.

Moore EE: Resuscitation and Evaluation of the Injured Patient, in Zuidema, Rutherford, and Ballinger (Eds). The Management of Trauma. WB Saunders Co., 1985; pp 1-26.

Thompson JS, Moore EE, Van Duzer-Moore S, et al: The Evolution of abdominal Stab Wound Management. Journal of Trauma 1980; 20: 478-484.

Anderson DW, McLaurin RL: The National Head and Spinal Cord Injury survey. Journal of Neurosurgery 1980; 53: S1-543.

Cooper PR (ed): Head Injury, ed 2. Baltimore, Williams and Wilkins, 1987.

Gennarelli TA: Emergency Department Management of Head Injuries. Emergency Medicine Clinics of North America 1984; 2: 749-760.

Jennett B, Teasdale G: Management of Head Injuries. Philadelphis, Davis, 1981.

Pitts LH: Neurological Evaluation of the Head Injury Patient. Clinical Neurosurgery 1982; 29: 203-224.

Light RW. Management of Spontaneous Pneumothorax. Am. Rev. Res. Dis. 1993; 148, 1: 245-248.

Light RW. Pneumothorax. In: Light RW, ed. Pleural Diseases. Philadelphis; Lea & Febiger, 1990; 237-62.

Mirvis SE. Imaging of Thoracic Trauma. In: Turney SZ, Rodriguez A, Cowley RA. Management of Cardiothoracic Trauma. Baltimore; Williams and Wilkins, 1990: 27-94.

HEMATOLOGY

By Cameron Dick, M.D.

TRANSFUSION REACTIONS

I. **Acute Hemolytic Transfusion Reaction:**
   A. **Clinical Presentation:** This rare reaction is most commonly associated with ABO incompatibility, and it is usually related to a clerical error. Early symptoms include sudden onset of anxiety, flushing, tachycardia, and hypotension. Chest and back pain, fever and dyspnea are common.
   B. Life threatening manifestations include vascular collapse (shock), renal failure, bronchospasm, and disseminated intravascular coagulation.
   C. Hemoglobinuria, and hemoglobinemia occurs found due to intravascular red cell lysis.
   D. A positive direct antiglobulin test (direct Coomb's test) will be found after transfusion. The severity of reaction is usually related to the volume of RBC's infused.
   E. **Management:**
      1. Discontinue transfusion and notify blood bank immediately. Send the unused donor blood and a sample of recipient's venous blood for retyping and repeat cross match including direct and indirect Coomb's test.
      2. Check urine analysis for free hemoglobin and check centrifuged plasma for pink coloration (indicating free hemoglobin).
      3. Manage hypotension with normal saline or plasma expanders. Vasopressors may be used if volume replacement alone is inadequate to maintain blood pressure. Central venous monitoring may be necessary.
      4. Maintain adequate renal perfusion with volume replacement as clinically indicated. Mannitol and/or furosemide may be used to maintain urine output after adequate volume replacement has been given.
      5. Monitor PT/PTT, platelets, fibrinogen, and fibrin degradation products for evidence of disseminated intravascular coagulation. Replace required clotting factors with fresh frozen plasma, platelets, and/or cryoprecipitate as indicated.
      6. In rare circumstances, exchange transfusions have been performed for massive intravascular hemolysis.

II. **Febrile Transfusion Reaction (nonhemolytic)**
   A. **Clinical Presentation:** This reaction occurs in 0.5-3% of transfusions, and is most commonly seen in patients receiving multiple transfusions. Clinically, chills develop followed by fever, usually during or within a few

hours of transfusion. This reaction may be severe but is usually mild and self limited.

B. **Management:**
1. Provide symptomatic and supportive care with acetaminophen and diphenhydramine. Meperidine 50 mg IV is useful in treating chills.
2. More serious transfusion reactions must be excluded.

III. **Transfusion Related Noncardiogenic Pulmonary Edema:**
A. **Clinical Presentation:** Sudden development of severe respiratory distress.
B. Associated with fever, chills, chest pain, and hypotension.
C. Chest radiograph demonstrates diffuse pulmonary edema. This reaction may be severe and life threatening but generally resolves within 48 hours.
D. **Management:**
1. Provide supportive measures for pulmonary edema and hypoxemia including mechanical ventilatory support and hemodynamic monitoring if needed.
2. Diuretics are useful only if fluid overload is present.

DISSEMINATED INTRAVASCULAR COAGULATION

I. **Clinical Manifestations:**
A. Generalized ecchymosis and petechiae, bleeding from peripheral IV sites, central catheters. surgical wounds, and oozing from gums are common presenting findings.
B. Gastrointestinal and urinary tract bleeding are frequently encountered. Grayish discoloration or cyanosis of the distal fingers, toes, or ears may be seen due to intravascular thrombosis.
C. Large, sharply demarcated ecchymotic areas may be seen as a result of thrombosis of the dermal blood supply.

II. **Diagnosis:**
A. **Laboratory Findings:** May be quite variable. No single parameter is diagnostic of DIC. Repeated testing of coagulation parameters may provide a kinetic assessment of the rate and degree of factor consumption or replacement.
B. **Peripheral Smear:** Evidence of microangiopathic hemolysis with schistocytes. Thrombocytopenia (a persistently normal platelet count nearly excludes the diagnosis of acute DIC).
C. **Coagulation Studies:** PT, PTT, and thrombin time are generally prolonged. Fibrinogen levels are depleted (<150 mg/dL). Fibrin

degradation products are elevated (>10 mg/dL). D-dimer is elevated (>0.5 mg/dL; sensitivity 85%, specificity 97%).

III. Management:

A. Treat the primary underlying precipitating condition (sepsis). Reversal of the syndrome depends on the treatment of the underlying disorder, despite efforts to replace coagulation factors and platelets,

B. Manage severe hemorrhage and shock with fluids and red blood cell transfusions.

C. **If the Patient Is at High Risk of Bleeding or Actively Bleeding with Biochemical Evidence of DIC:** Replace fibrinogen, platelets, and clotting factors with cryoprecipitate, fresh frozen plasma, and platelets as appropriate.

D. **If Factor Replacement Therapy Is Transfused:** Fibrinogen and platelet levels should be obtained 30-60 minutes post-transfusion and every 4-6 hours thereafter to determine the efficacy of therapy, and to determine need for successive infusions. Each unit of platelets should increase platelet count by 5000-10,000/mcL. Each unit of cryoprecipitate should increase fibrinogen by an increment of 5-10 mg/dL.

E. **Heparin:**

1. The use of heparin is controversial. Indications include evidence of fibrin deposition (i.e. dermal necrosis, acral ischemia, venous thromboembolism).

2. Consider use when the coagulopathy is believed to be secondary to any of the following primary conditions: Retained dead fetus, amniotic fluid embolus, giant hemangiomas, aortic aneurysm, solid tumors, promyelocytic leukemia. Also consider heparin when clotting factors cannot be corrected with replacement therapy alone.

3. If heparin therapy is used, the dosage and route of administration should be tailored to the underlying disorder. Generally, heparin therapy is initiated at a relatively low dose (5-10 U/kg/hr) by continuous IV infusion without bolus. Coagulation parameters must then be followed to guide therapy. If desired increments of clotting factors are not obtained, then heparin dose may be increased by 2.5 U/kg/hr until desired effect.

THROMBOLYTIC ASSOCIATED BLEEDING

I. Clinical Presentation:

A. Post-fibrinolysis hemorrhage has varied presentations, ranging from a sudden neurologic deficit (intracranial bleeding) to massive volume loss (as in GI bleeding) to a gradual decline in hemoglobin without overt evidence of bleeding.

B. Occult sources of blood loss must always be considered, such as into the retroperitoneal space, into the thigh (often related to femoral venous or arterial puncture), or into the peritoneum or thorax.

II. Laboratory Evaluation:

A. Elevated thrombin time and PTT identify a persistent lytic state; however, both are prolonged in the presence of heparin.

B. Prolonged reptilase time identifies the persistent lytic state in the presence of heparin.

C. Depleted fibrinogen in the fibrinolytic state will be reflected by the elevated PTT, thrombin time, or reptilase time. Post-transfusion fibrinogen levels is a useful indicator of response to replacement therapy.

D. Elevated fibrin degradation products confirm the presence of a lytic state.

E. The bleeding time as an indicator of platelet function may be a helpful guide to platelet replacement therapy if the patient has persistent bleeding despite factor replacement with cryoprecipitate, and fresh frozen plasma.

III. Management:

A. Discontinue thrombolytics, aspirin, and heparin immediately, and consider protamine reversal of heparin.

B. Place two large bore IV catheters for volume replacement. If possible, apply local pressure to bleeding sites.

C. Send blood specimens for PT/PTT, fibrinogen, and thrombin time. Check reptilase time if patient is also receiving heparin.

D. Patient's blood type should be typed and crossed because urgent transfusion may be needed.

E. **Transfusion:**

1. Cryoprecipitate (10 units over 10 minutes) should be transfused as a first-line measure to correct the lytic state. Transfusions may be repeated until fibrinogen level is above 100 mg/dL or hemostasis is achieved.

2. Fresh frozen plasma transfusion is also important for replacement of factor VIII and V. Depending on the extent of hemorrhage, caution must be used during transfusion therapy to avoid volume overload. If bleeding persists after cryoprecipitate and FFP replacement, check a bleeding time and consider platelet transfusion if bleeding time is greater than 9 minutes. if bleeding time is less than 9 minutes, then antifibrinolytic drugs may be warranted.

F. **Antifibrinolytic Agents:**

1. Aminocaproic acid (EACA) inhibits the binding of plasmin to fibrin and plasminogen to fibrinogen. Consider using when replacement of blood products are not sufficient to attain hemostasis; potential risk of serious thrombotic complications.

2. loading dose: 5 g or 0.1 g/kg IV infused in 250 cc NS over 30-60 min, followed by continuous infusion at 0.5 to 1.0 g/h until bleeding is controlled. Use with caution in upper urinary tract bleeding due to the potential for obstruction. Contraindicated in DIC.

G. **If Bleeding Is Suspected on the Basis of Falling Hemoglobin Without Overt Evidence of Blood Loss:** Occult sources must be considered including the retroperitoneal space, thigh (often related to femoral venous or arterial puncture), bleeding into other body cavities (peritoneum, thorax).

ANTICOAGULANT OVERDOSE

I. **HEPARIN OVERDOSE:**

A. Protamine Sulfate forms a heparin-protamine complex and reverses the anticoagulant effect of heparin. Protamine neutralizes heparin within 5 minutes.

B. Indication-Protamine should be considered if heparin was given within 4 hours of the onset of bleeding. The plasma half-life of heparin is 1-2 hours and protamine is unlikely to be beneficial more than 4 hours after last heparin dose.

C. **Dosing:**
   1. **Recent Heparin Bolus**: 1 mg protamine sulfate IV for each 100 units of heparin administered.
   2. **Continuous Heparin Infusion:** 1 mg protamine sulfate IV for each 100 units given over the preceding 4 hours.
   3. **If Heparin Has Been Discontinued for More than 30 Min:** Reduce protamine dosage by 50%.
   4. Doses should be infused slowly over 1-3 minutes and should not exceed 50 mg in any 10 minute period.

D. **Adverse effects:** Mild hypotension; anaphylactic reactions are uncommon. Risk for allergic reactions in diabetic patients exposed to protamine through some insulin preparations.

II. **WARFARIN OVERDOSE:**

A. **Elimination Measures:** Gastric lavage and activated charcoal if recent oral ingestion of warfarin (Coumadin).

B. **Reversal of Coumadin Anticoagulation:** Coagulopathy may be corrected rapidly or slowly depending on the following factors: 1)Intensity of hypocoagulability, 2) severity or risk of bleeding, 3) need for reinstitution of anticoagulation.

C. **Emergent Reversal:**
   1. Fresh frozen plasma: Replace Vitamin K dependent factors with FFP 15-20 mL/kg followed by 5-7 mL/kg every 8-12 hours.
   2. Vitamin K 25 mg in 50 cc NS to infuse no faster than 1 mg/min; risk of anaphylactoid reactions and shock; slow infusion minimizes risk.

D. **Reversal over 24-48 Hours:** Vitamin K 10-25 mg subcutaneously. Full reversal of anticoagulation will result in resistance to further Coumadin therapy for several days.

E. **Temporary Correction:** Lower doses of Vitamin K (0.5-1.0 mg) will lower prothrombin time without interfering with reinitiation of Coumadin.

References

Lee GR, Bithell TC, Foerster J, Athens JW, Lukens JN: Wintrobe's Clinical Hematology, 9th Ed. Lea an Febiger, 1992, pp.652-687, 1480-1490.

Rippe JM, Irwin RS, Alpert JS, Fink MP: Intensive Care Medicine, 2nd Ed. Little, Brown and Co., 1991, pp.1019-1021, 1055-1061.

Carr JM, McKinney M, McDonagh J: Diagnosis of Disseminated Intravascular Coagulation, Role of D-Dimer. Am J Clin Pathol 1989;91:280-287.

Feinstein DI: Treatment of Disseminated Intravascular Coagulation. Seminars in Thrombosis and Hemostasis. 1988;14:351-362.

Sane DC, Califf RM, Topol EJ, Stump DC, Mark DB, Greenberg CS: Bleeding during Thrombolytic Therapy for Acute Myocardial Infarction: Mechanisms and Management. Ann of Int Med. 1989;111:1010-1022.

INFECTIOUS DISEASES

By S. Salman J. Naqvi, M.D.,M.Sc.

EMPIRIC THERAPY OF MENINGITIS

I. **Labs:** CBC, SMA 12. Blood C&S x 2. UA with micro, urine C&S. Stool, throat, nasal C&S. Antibiotic levels peak & trough after 3rd dose.

   CSF Tube 1-Gram stain of fluid or sediment (if fluid is clear), C&S for bacteria (1-4 mL).

   CSF Tube 2-Cell count & differential (1-2 mL).

   CSF Tube 3-Glucose, protein (1-2 mL).

   CSF Tube 4-Latex agglutination or counterimmunoelectrophoresis antigen tests for S. pneumoniae, H. influenzae (type B), N. meningitides, E. coli, group B strep, cryptococcus, viral cultures, VDRL (8-10 mL).

   Other Tests: CXR, ECG, PPD with controls.

II. **Treatment:**

   A. Acute bacterial meningitis is a medical emergency.

   B. If mass lesion not suspected: Complete lumbar puncture before CT scan or MRI, then initiate antibiotics.

   C. If mass lesion suspected (subacute development of symptoms suggest mass lesion): initiate antibiotics before CT scan or MRI; perform lumbar puncture if no signs of elevated intracranial pressure.

   D. **Meningitis Empiric Therapy 15-50 years old**

   -Ampicillin 2 gm IV q4h (with 3rd gen cephalosporin) **AND EITHER**
   Ceftriaxone (Rocephin) 2 gm IV q12h (max 4 gm/d) **OR**
   Cefotaxime (Claforan) 2 gm IV q4h **OR**
   Ceftizoxime (Cefizox) 2 gm IV q4h **OR**
   Ceftazidime (Fortaz) 2 gm IV q4h
   -Consider dexamethasone IV.

   E. **Empiric Therapy >50 years old, Alcoholic, Corticosteroids or Hematologic malignancy or other Debilitating Condition:**

   -Ampicillin 2 gm IV q4h or penicillin G **AND EITHER**
   Cefotaxime (Claforan) 2 gm IV q4h **OR**
   Ceftriaxone (Rocephin) 2 gm IV q12h (max 4 g/d) **OR**
   Ceftizoxime (Cefizox) 2 gm IV q4h **OR**
   Ceftazidime (Fortaz) 2 gm IV q4h
   -Consider dexamethasone IV.

   F. **Post-Neurosurgical Procedure or Post-Cranial Spinal Trauma:**

   -Vancomycin 2 gm IV q6-8h, **AND**
   -Ceftazidime (Fortaz) 2 gm IV q8h, (max 12 g/d)

CEREBRAL SPINAL FLUID ANALYSIS

DISEASE	COLOR	PROTEIN	CELLS	SUGAR
Normal CSF Fluid	Clear	<50 mg/100 mL	<5 lymphs/mm^3	>40 mg/100 mL, ½-2/3 blood sugar drawn at same time
Bacterial meningitis early viral or tuberculous meningitis	Yellow opalescent	Elevated 50-1500	25-10000 WBC with predominate polys	low
Tuberculous, fungal, partially treated bacterial, syphilitic meningitis, meningeal metastases	Clear opalescent	Elevated usually <500	10-500 WBC with predominant lymphs	20-40, low
Viral meningitis, partially treated bacterial meningitis, & encephalitis, toxoplasmosis, parameningeal infection	Clear opalescent	Slightly elevated or normal	10-500 WBC with predominant lymphs	normal, may be low

EMPIRIC TREATMENT OF PNEUMONIA

Laboratory Evaluation:
A. CBC with differential; SMA 12, ABG. Blood C&S x 2. Sputum Gram stain, C&S. UA. Titers for mycoplasma, legionella, coccidiomycosis.
B. CXR PA, LAT, ECG, PPD.

Treatment:
A. Oxygen by NC at 2-4 L/min or 24-50% Venti-mask or 100% non-rebreather (reservoir); titrate to keep O_2 sat >90%.
B. Pulse oximeter, I&O, nasotracheal suctioning prn, incentive spirometry.
C. **Community Acquired Pneumonia 5-40 Years Old Without Underlying Lung Disease:**
   -Erythromycin (Eramycin) 500 mg IV qid **OR**
   -Cefuroxime 25 mg/kg IV q8h (children) or 0.75-1.5 gm IV q8h (adults) **OR**
   -Ampicillin/sulbactam (Unasyn) 1.5-3.0 gm IV q6h.
   -Clarithromycin (Biaxin) 250-500 mg PO bid 7-10 days **OR**
   -Azithromycin (Zithromax) 500 mg PO x 1, then 250 mg PO qd x 4 days (T½ 60 hours). **OR**
D. **Community Acquired Pneumonia >40 years old:**
   -Erythromycin 500 mg IV q6h **OR**
   -Cefuroxime (Zinacef) 1.5 gm IV q8h **OR**
   -Cefotaxime (Claforan) 1-2 gm IV q8 **OR**
   -Ceftriaxone (Rocephin) 1-2 gm IV q12h **OR**
   -Trimethoprim/Sulfamethoxazole (Septra DS) 6-10 mg TMP/kg/d IV in 2-3 divided doses **OR**
   -Ampicillin/Sulbactam (Unasyn) 1.5 gm IV q6h.
E. **COPD with Pneumonia:**
   -Erythromycin 500 mg IV q6h **AND/OR**
   -Cefuroxime axetil (Ceftin) 250-500 mg PO bid **OR**
   -Cefotaxime (Claforan) 1-2 gm IV q4-6h **OR**
   -Ceftriaxone (Rocephin) 1-2 gm IV q12h **OR**
   -Ceftizoxime (Cefizox) 1-2 gm IV q8-12h **OR**
   -Cefuroxime (Zinacef) 0.75-1.5 gm IV q8h **OR**
   -Ampicillin/sulbactam (Unasyn) 1.5-3 gm IV q6h **OR**
   -Amoxicillin/clavulanate (Augmentin) 250-500 mg PO q8h **OR**
   -Piperacillin/tazobactam (Zosyn) 3.375 gm IV q6h **OR**
   -Ticarcillin/clavulanate (Timentin) 3.1 gm IV q4-6h (200-300 mg/kg/d).
F. **Alcoholics, Diabetics, Heart Failure, Debilitated or other Underlying Diseases:**
   -Erythromycin 0.5-1.0 gm IV q6h **AND EITHER**
   Cefotaxime (Claforan) 1-2 gm IV q4-6h **OR**
   Ceftriaxone (Rocephin) 1-2 gm IV q12h **OR**

Cefuroxime (Zinacef) 0.75-1.5 gm IV q8h **OR**

Ceftizoxime (Cefizox) 1-2 gm IV q8 **OR**

TMP/SMX IV 6-10 mg TMP/Kg per day in 2-3 divided doses **OR**

Ampicillin/Sulbactam (Unasyn) 1.5-3 gm IV q6h. **OR**

-Piperacillin/tazobactam (Zosyn) 3.375 gm IV q6h; not adequate coverage for pseudomonas **OR**

-Ticarcillin/clavulanate Timentin 3.1 gm IV q4-6h (200-300 mg/Kg/day).

G. **Nosocomial, Hospital Acquired, Broad Spectrum Antibiotic Associated Pneumonia:**
-Tobramycin 80-100 mg IV q8h (3-5 mg/kg/d) **AND EITHER**
Ceftriaxone 1-2 gm IV q12-24h **OR**
Ceftizoxime (Cefizox) or other 3rd generation cephalosporin (see above) **OR**
Piperacillin, Azlocillin, Mezlocillin or Ticarcillin 3 gm IV q4-6h (with tobramycin or gentamicin) **OR**
Imipenem/cilastatin (Primaxin) 0.5-1.0 gm IV q6-8h.

H. **Aspiration Pneumonia (community acquired):**
-Clindamycin (Cleocin) 600-900 mg IV q8h (with or without gentamicin or 3rd gen cephalosporin) **OR**
-Ampicillin/Sulbactam (Unasyn) 1.5-3 gm IV q6h (with or without gentamicin or 3rd gen cephalosporin) **OR**
-Ticarcillin/Clavulanic acid (Timentin) 3.1 gm IV q4-6h (with or without Gentamicin) **OR**
-Piperacillin/tazobactam (Zosyn) 3.375 gm IV q6h **OR**
-Imipenem/Cilastatin (Primaxin)0.5-1.0 gm IV q6-8h

I. **Aspiration Pneumonia (nosocomial):**
-Tobramycin 2 mg/kg IV then 1.7 mg/kg IV q8h **OR**
-Ceftazidime 1-2 gm IV q8h **AND EITHER**
Clindamycin (Cleocin) 600-900 mg IV q8h **OR**
Penicillin G 1-2 MU IV q4h **OR**
-Ticarcillin/clavulanate, or Imipenem/cilastatin (see above)

J. **Bacterial Pneumonia Complicating Influenza Tracheobronchitis:**
-Nafcillin (Nafcil) 1-2 gm IV q4h **OR**
-Oxacillin (Bactocill) 1-2 gm IV q4h
-Vancomycin (Vancocin) 1 gm IV q12h ; use if allergic to penicillin.
-If H Influenza use prevalent Unasyn, Timentin or Imipenem.

K. **Alcoholics, Overdose, Cerebrovascular Events (Aspiration prone):**
-Clindamycin 150-900 mg IV/IM q8h **OR**
-Penicillin 10-12 million units daily in divided doses **OR**
-Ticarcillin/Clavulanate (Timentin) 3.1 gm IV q6h (200-300 mg/kg/d) **OR**
-Ampicillin/Sulbactam (Unasyn) 1.5 gm IV q6h **OR**
-Piperacillin/tazobactam (Zosyn) 3.375 gm IV q6h **OR**

-Imipenem 0.5-1 gm IV q6h over 30 min.

PNEUMOCYSTIS CARINII PNEUMONIA IN PATIENTS WITH AIDS

Laboratory Evaluation:
A. ABG, CBC, SMA 18. Blood C&S x 2 for bacterial, fungal culture. Sputum for Gram stain, C&S, AFB. Sputum stain for Pneumocystis. Induce sputum with nebulized 3% saline after gargling with 3% saline.
B. Serum CD4 lymphocyte count, VDRL, hepatitis B surface antigen, anti-HBs, titers for toxoplasmosis. UA. CXR PA & LAT.

Bronchoscopic Considerations: Consider bronchoscopic diagnosis if sputum non-diagnostic or CXR not typical for PCP, or if patient not responding to empiric therapy.

Treatment:
Pneumocystis Carinii Pneumonia Initial Therapy:
-Oxygen by NC at 2-4 L/min or by mask.
-Trimethoprim/sulfamethoxazole (Bactrim, Septra) 15-20 mg/kg/day (based on TMP) PO or IV in 3-4 divided doses x 21 days; TMP-SMX is the drug of choice.
-If moderately severe PCP (Pa02 <70 mm Hg): Give methylprednisolone 40 mg IV q8h or prednisone 40 mg PO bid for 5 days. Taper dose to one-half this amount for the next 5 days; then 20 mg qd until the end of antimicrobial therapy **OR**
-Pentamidine (Pentam) 3-4 mg/kg IV qd x 21 days, with methylprednisolone as above. Pentamidine is an alternate treatment if inadequate response to TMP-SMX.
-Atovaquone (Mepron) 750 mg PO tid x 21 days. Use restricted to those with mild to moderate PCP who are refractory to or intolerant of TMP-SMX.

Antiviral Therapy:
-Zidovudine (Retrovir)(CD4 <500, symptomatic AIDS)100 mg PO q4 hours or 100 mg five times a day; some physicians prescribe 200 mg tid. Dosage may be reduced to 100 mg tid if side effects are intolerable, or if significant anemia [100-mg caps] **OR**
-Didanosine (DDI, Videx) 200 mg PO bid for patients >60 kg; or 125 mg PO bid for patients <60 kg [100-mg, 150-mg buffered tablet may be mixed with water and taken on an empty stomach] **OR**
-Zalcitabine (DDC, Hivid) 0.375-0.75 mg PO q8h [0.375, 0.75 mg].
-Hold antiviral therapy during TMP/SMX therapy because of the marrow suppressing side effects of both drugs combined

OPPORTUNISTIC INFECTIONS IN PATIENTS WITH AIDS

Oral Candidiasis:
- Fluconazole (Diflucan) Acute: 100-200 mg po qd; higher dosages might be necessary. Maintenance: 100-200 mg po once weekly or 50-100 mg po qd **OR**
- Ketoconazole (Nizoral), acute: 400 mg po qd 1-2 weeks or until resolved. Maintenance: 200 mg po qd-bid for 7 consecutive days per month or qd if necessary. **OR**
- Clotrimazole (Mycelex) troches 10 mg dissolved slowly in mouth 5 times/d **OR**
- Nystatin (Mycostatin) 100,000 U/mL, swish and swallow 5 mL po q 6 hr or one 500,000-unit tablet dissolved slowly in mouth q6h.

Candida Esophagitis:
- Fluconazole 200-400 mg po qd x 14-21 days; higher dosages might be required **OR**
- Ketoconazole 200 mg po bid.
- Maintenance with fluconazole (100 mg po qd) or ketoconazole (200 mg PO qd) may be required at the lowest effective dose.

Primary or Recurrent Mucocutaneous HSV
- Acyclovir (Zovirax), 200-400 mg po 5 times a day for 10 days, or 5 mg/kg IV q8h OR In cases of acyclovir resistance, foscarnet, 40 mg/kg IV q8h, via infusion pump only, for 21 days.
- Prophylaxis: Acyclovir (Zovirax) 400 mg PO bid.

Herpes Simplex Encephalitis:
- Acyclovir 10 mg/kg IV q8h x 10-21 days.

Herpes Varicella Zoster
- Acyclovir 10 mg/kg IV over 60 min q8h for 7-14 days **OR** 800 mg PO 5 times/d x 7-10 days.

Cytomegalovirus infections:
- Ganciclovir (Cytovene) 5 mg/kg IV (dilute in 100 mLs D5W over 60 min) q12h x 14-21 days for retinitis, colitis, esophagitis (concurrent use with zidovudine may increase hematological toxicity)

Suppressive Treatment for CMV:
- Ganciclovir 5 mg/kg IV qd, or 6 mg/kg 5 times/wk.

Toxoplasmosis:
- Clindamycin 600-900 mg po or IV qid plus pyrimethamine 25-75 mg po qd-qOD plus leucovorin calcium (folinic acid) 10-25 mg po qd for 6-8 weeks for acute therapy; lifetime suppression with highest tolerated dosage.

Suppressive Treatment for Toxoplasmosis:
- Pyrimethamine 25-50 mg PO qd with or without sulfadiazine 0.5-1.0 Gm PO q6h; and folinic acid 5-10 mg PO qd. **OR**
- Pyrimethamine 50 mg PO qd; and clindamycin 300 mg PO q6h; and folinic acid 5-10 mg PO qd.

Cryptococcus Neoformans Meningitis:
- Amphotericin B 0.7-1.0 mg/kg/d IV; amphotericin total dosage not to exceed 2 g, with or without 5-flucytosine 100 mg/kg po qd in in divided doses for first 2-4 weeks or until clinically improved, followed by fluconazole 400 mg po qd or itraconazole 200 mg po bid 6-8 weeks

  OR
- Fluconazole 400-800 mg po qd for 8-12 weeks

Suppressive Treatment for Cryptococcus:
- Fluconazole (Diflucan) 200 mg PO qd indefinitely.

Active Tuberculosis:
- Isoniazid (INH) 300 mg PO qd; and rifampin 600 mg PO qd; and pyrazinamide 15-25 mg/kg PO qd; and ethambutol 15-25 mg/kg PO qd; or streptomycin 15 mg/kg IM qd, or 20 mg/kg IM twice/wk.
- Pyridoxine (Vitamin B6) 50 mg PO qd concurrent with INH.
- All four drugs are continued for 2 months; isoniazid and rifampin (depending on susceptibility testing) are continued for a period of at least 9 months and at least 6 months after the last negative cultures.

Disseminated Mycobacterium Avium Complex (MAC):
- Clarithromycin (Biaxin) 500-1000 mg PO bid; or Azithromycin (Zithromax) 500 mg PO qd; **AND EITHER**

  Ethambutol 15-25 mg/kg PO qd, **OR**

  Clofazimine (Lamprene) 100-200 mg PO qd, **OR**

  Ciprofloxacin (Cipro) 750 mg PO bid or 400 mg IV bid.

Prophylaxis for MAC:
- Rifabutin (Mycobutin), 300 mg PO qd or 150 mg PO bid.

Disseminated Coccidioidomycosis:
- Amphotericin B 0.5-0.8 mg/kg IV qd, until total dose 2.0-2.5 gms. **OR**
- Fluconazole (Diflucan) 400-800 mg PO and/or IV qd.

Disseminated Histoplasmosis:
- Amphotericin B 0.5-0.8 mg/kg IV qd, until total dose 15 mg/kg. **OR**
- Itraconazole (Sporanox) 200 mg PO bid.
- AIDS associated diarrhea-see page 62

Suppressive Treatment for Histoplasmosis:
- Itraconazole (Sporanox) 200 mg PO bid **OR**
- Amphotericin B 0.5-0.8 mg/kg IV q/wk.

SEPTIC SHOCK

Labs: CBC with differential, SMA 7 & 12, blood C&S x 3, PT/PTT. UA with micro. Cultures of urine, sputum, wound, IV catheters, ascitic fluid, decubitus ulcers, pleural fluid.

Consider: CXR, KUB, sinus films, ECG, Indium/Gallium scan, ultrasound, consider lumbar puncture.

Treatment:

-Oxygen at 2-5 L/min by NC or mask or mechanical ventilation if indicated.

Non-immunocompromised Adults, Antibiotics: if pelvic or intra-abdominal infection, use ampicillin with gentamicin/tobramycin, add clindamycin or metronidazole ; **OR** use cefoxitin & gent/tobramycin **OR** Unasyn & gent/tobramycin).   May use 3rd generation cephalosporins in place of aminoglycosides if resistant gram-neg pathogens not suspected.

-Ceftazidime (Fortaz) 1-2 g IV q8h **OR**

-Ceftizoxime (Cefizox) 1-2 gm IV q8h **OR**

-Cefotaxime (Claforan) 2 gm q4-6h **OR**

-Ceftriaxone (Rocephin) 1-2 gm IV q12h (max 4 gm/d). **OR**

-Cefoxitin (Mefoxin) 1-2 gms q6-8h **OR**

-Cefotetan (Cefotan) 1-2 Gms IV q12h **OR**

-Ampicillin 2 gm IV q4h **OR**

-Piperacillin, ticarcillin or mezlocillin 3 gms IV q4-6h **AND**

-Gentamicin or tobramycin 100-120 mg (1.5-2 mg/kg) IV, then 80 mg IV q8h (3-5 mg/kg/d) **AND**

-Clindamycin 600-900 IV q8h (15-30 mg/kg/d) **OR**

-Metronidazole 500 mg (7.5 mg/kg) IV q6h **OR**

-Piperacillin/tazobactam (Zosyn) 3.375 gm IV q6h **OR**

-Ticarcillin/clavulanic acid (Timentin) 3.1 gm IV q4-6h (200-300 mg/kg/d) (with gent/tobramycin). **OR**

-Ampicillin/Sulbactam (Unasyn) 1.5-3.0 gm IV q6h (with gent/tobramycin) **OR**

-Imipenem/cilastatin (Primaxin) 0.5-1.0 gm IV q6-8h (with gent/tobramycin).

-Vancomycin 500 mg IV q6h or 1 gm IV q12h; use if allergy to penicillin or if resistant pathogens are present.

Nosocomial sepsis with IV catheter or IV drug abuse

-Nafcillin or oxacillin 2 gms IV q4h **AND**

Gentamicin or Tobramycin as above; **AND EITHER**

Ceftazidime or Ceftizoxime 1-2 gms IV q8h **OR**

Piperacillin, ticarcillin or mezlocillin 3 gm IV q4-6h.

-Vancomycin 1 gm IV q12h; if allergic to penicillin or if resistant pathogens are present.

CANDIDA SEPTICEMIA:
   -Amphotericin B, 1 mg test dose (D5W 100 mLs 60 min), then 10-20 mg
      (D5W 250 mLs over 3-4h) the same day, then 0.4-0.5 mg/Kg/day (D5W
      250-500 mLs over 4-6h); total dose 0.5-1.0 gm.
Blood Pressure Support: Use colloids or crystalloids as indicated.   If
   nonresponsive, use dopamine and dobutamine.

PERITONITIS

Labs: CBC with differential, SMA 12, albumin, LDH, amylase, lactate. PT/PTT,
   UA with micro, C&S.
PARACENTESIS
TUBE 1 - Cell count & differential (1-2 mL, EDTA purple top tube)
TUBE 2 - Gram stain of sediment, C&S, AFB, fungal C&S (3-4 mL); inject 10-20
   mL into anaerobic & aerobic culture bottle.
TUBE 3 - Glucose, protein, albumin, LDH, triglyceride, specific gravity, bilirubin,
   amylase, fibrinogen, (2-3 mL, red top tube).
SYRINGE - pH, lactate (3 mL).
Note:. Serum/fluid albumin gradient should be determined.
Other Tests: Cytology, plain film of abdomen.
CXR PA & LAT, ECG, abdominal ultrasound.
Treatment:
Spontaneous Bacterial Peritonitis (nephrotic or cirrhotic):
Option 1:
   -Ampicillin * 1-2 gms IV q 4-6h; **AND EITHER**
   Cefotaxime (Claforan) 1-2 gm IV q4-6h **OR**
   Ceftizoxime (Cefizox) 1-2 gms IV q8h **OR**
   Gentamicin or Tobramycin 1.5 mg/Kg IV, then 1 mg/Kg q8h (adjust for renal
      function).
Option 2:
   -Ticarcillin/clavulanate (Timentin) 3.1 gms IV q6h **OR**
   -Piperacillin/tazobactam (Zosyn) 3.375 gm IV q6h
Option 3:
   -Imipenem/cilastatin (Primaxin) 0.5-1.0 gm IV q6h.
*Vancomycin 500 mg IV q6h or 1 gm IV q12h if penicillin allergic.
Secondary Bacterial Peritonitis:
Option 1:
   -Cefoxitin (Mefoxin) 2 gm IV q6-8h **OR**
   -Ampicillin 1-2 gm IV q4-6h **AND**

Gentamicin or tobramycin (aminoglycosides are not recommended in cirrhotics) 100-120 mg (1.5 mg/kg); then 80 mg IV q8h (5 mg/kg/d)(if resistant, use amikacin) **AND**

Metronidazole 500 mg IV q6h (15-30 mg/kg/d)

Option 2:

-Piperacillin/tazobactam (Zosyn) 3.375 gm IV q6h with an aminoglycoside as above **OR**

-Ticarcillin/clavulanic acid (Timentin) 3.1 gm IV q4-6h (200-300 mg/kg/d) with aminoglycoside as above.

Option 3:

-Ampicillin/Sulbactam (Unasyn) 1.5-3.0 gm IV q6h with aminoglycoside as above.

Option 4:

-Imipenem/cilastatin (Primaxin) 0.5-1.0 gm IV q6-8h.

Peritonitis Associated with Ambulatory Peritoneal Dialysis:

-Tobramycin 70-140 mg/2 L bag initially then 8-16 mg/2 L maintenance **AND/OR**

-Vancomycin 1000-1200 mg/2 L initially then 30-50 mg/2 L maintenance.

Fungal:

-Amphotericin B (2 mg/L 1st 24 hours then 1.5 mg/L) **AND**

Flucytosine (100 mg/L 1st 3 days then 30 mg/L)

Symptomatic Meds:

-Ranitidine (Zantac) 50 mg IV q8h or 150 mg PO bid; in azotemic patients adjust dose to 50 mg IV q24h or 150 mg PO qhs.

-Acetaminophen 325 mg PO q4-6h prn temp >101.

TOXIC SHOCK SYNDROME

Labs: CBC with differential, SMA 7 & 12, calcium, Mg, CPK isoenzymes, blood C&S x 2, UA with micro, C&S, PT/PTT, thrombin time, fibrinogen, fibrin degradation products, lactate, ABG.

Treatment:

-Volume replacement with normal saline or Ringers lactate until hemodynamically stable.

-Surgical therapy for localized infection.

-Nafcillin or Oxacillin 2 gm IV q4h x 10 days **OR**

-Vancomycin (if penicillin allergic) 500 mg IV q6h or 1 gm IV q12h.

VANCOMYCIN THERAPY

I. **CDC Recommendations for Prevention and Control of Vancomycin-Resistant Enterococci:** The following guidelines have been developed due to increasing reports of emergence of vancomycin-resistant enterococci (VRE), vancomycin-resistant S. aureus (VRSA) and vancomycin-resistant S. epidermidis (VRSE).

 A. **Appropriate or Acceptable Vancomycin Use:**
   1. Treatment of serious infections due to beta-lactam resistant gram-positive pathogens.
   2. Treatment of infections due to gram-positive pathogens in patients with a serious allergy to beta-lactam antibiotics.
   3. Severe and potentially life-threatening antibiotic-associated colitis (AAC), or recurrent AAC previously treated with metronidazole.
   4. Endocarditis prophylaxis as recommended by the American Heart Association.
   5. Surgical prophylaxis involving implantation of prosthetic devices at institutions with high incidence of infections due to methicillin-resistant S. aureus and/or S. Epidermidis. A single dose is administered just prior to surgery followed by a maximum of two doses post-operatively.

II. **Treatment of Vancomycin-Resistant Enterococcal Infections:**
 A. Chloramphenicol 500-1000 mg IV q6h. Monitor CBC, reticulocyte count, and serum chloramphenicol levels.

REFERENCES

AIDS:
1- Hughes W.T. Opportunistic Infections in AIDS Patients. Opportunistic Infections 95:81-93, 1994
2- Lane HCLaughon B.E. Falloon J., et. al. Recent Advances in the Management of AIDS-related Opportunistic Infections. Ann. Intern. Med. 120:945-955, 1994.
Meningitis:
1- Tunkel A.R, Wispelway B, Scheld W.N: Bacterial meningitis; Recent advances in pathophysiology and treatment. Ann Int Med 112:610,1990.
2- Viladrich P.F, Gudiol F, Linares R, et al: Characteristic and antibiotic therapy of adult meningitis due to penicillin-resistant pneumococci, Am J Med 84:839, 1988.
3- Buckwold F.J, Hand R, Hansebout R.R: Hospital-acquired bacterial meningitis in neurosurgical patients. J neurosurg 46:494, 1977.
4- Label M.H, Fray B.J, Syrogiannopoulos G.A, et al: Dexamethasone therapy for bacterial meningitis. Results of double-blinded, placebo-controlled trials. N Eng J Med 319:964. 1988.

5- Gaunt P.N, Lambert B.E: Single-dose Ciprofloxicin for eradication of pharyngeal carriage of Neisseria meningitides. J Antimicrob Chemother 21:489. 1988.

6-Sanford J.P: The Sanford guide to antimicrobial therapy p3-5. 1993.

Pneumonia:

1-Pachon J, et al: Severe community acquired pneumonia. Am Rev Respir Dis 142:36973, 1990

2-Fong G D et al: New and emerging etiologies for community acquired pneumonia with implications of therapy: a prospective multicenter study of 359 cases. Medicine 69:307-16, 1990

Vancomycin Resistance:

1-California Department of Health Services. Part I. A new threat to health care facilities in California: vancomycin resistant enterococci. California Morbidity, April 22, 1994, #31/32.

2-Centers for Disease Control and Prevention. Preventing the spread of vancomycin resistance-report from the hospital infection control practices advisory committee. 59 Fed Reg 1995;25:757.

3-Edmond MB, Ober JF, Weinbaum DL, et al: Vancomycin-resistant enterococcal faecum bacteria: risk factor for infection. Clinical Infectious Diseases 1995; 20:1126-1133.

4-Noris AH, Reilly JP, Edelstein PH, et al: Chloramphenical for the treatment of vancomycin-resistant enterococcal infections. Clinical Infectious Diseases 1995; 20:1137-1144.

GASTROENTEROLOGY

By Theodore Shankel, MD

GASTROINTESTINAL BLEEDING

Labs: CBC, platelets, SMA 12, alkaline phosphatase, LDH, amylase, bilirubin, lactate, salicylate level, PT/PTT, type & cross for 3-8 U PRBC & 2-4 U FFP. Repeat CBC q6h x 24h. Portable CXR, upright abdomen, ECG. Surgery & gastroenterology consults.

Upper GI Bleeds: Endoscopy with possible coagulation or sclerotherapy; Sengstaken-Blakemore or Minnesota tube for tamponade. Consider intubation for patients with hemodynamically unstable GI bleeding.

Lower GI Bleeds: Sigmoidoscopy/colonoscopy, technetium 99m RBC scan, angiography with possible embolization.

General Measures:

1. A nasogastric tube should be inserted in all patients with a GI bleed, if the gastric aspirate is clear. Place a double lumen or single lumen nasogastric tube, then lavage with 2 L of room temperature saline, then connect low intermittent suction, repeat lavage q1h. Record volume & character of lavage.
2. Foley to closed drainage; I&O. Record stool character. Pulse oximeter. Place patient NPO.
3. **IV Fluids:** Minimum of two 16 gauge IV lines. 1-3 L NS IV wide open or over 1-3 hours.
4. As soon as available, transfuse PRBC's, to run as fast as possible, use blood loss rate and vital signs to guide transfusion rate. The hemoglobin and hematocrit may lag behind the clinical picture because of time required to equilibrate. Consider central venous pressure monitoring.
5. Oxygen 2-5 L by NC.

Medications:

-Ranitidine (Zantac) 50 mg IV bolus, then continuous infusion at 6.25-12.5 mg/h [150-300 mg in 500 mL D5W over 24h (21 cc/h)], or 50 mg IV q6-8h, followed by 150 mg PO bid **OR**

-Cimetidine (Tagamet) 300 mg IV bolus, then continuous infusion at 37.5-50 mg/h (900 mg in 500 cc D5W over 24h), or 300 mg IV q6-8h, followed by 300 mg PO tid-qid **OR**

-Famotidine (Pepcid) 20 mg IV q12h, followed by 20 mg PO q12h

Acute Variceal Hemorrhage:

-Vasopressin 20 U IV over 20-30 minutes, then 0.2-0.6 U/min [100 U in 250 mL of D5W (0.4 U/mL)], for 30 min, followed by increases of 0.2 U/min until bleeding stops or max of 1.0 U/min. If bleeding stops, taper over 24-

48h. Patient must be observed for arrhythmias, sinus bradycardia, hypertension, and angina **AND**

-Nitropaste (with vasopressin) 1 inch q6h **OR**

-Octreotide acetate (Sandostatin) 50 mcg IV over 5-10 min, followed by 50 mcg/hr IV infusion x 48h (1200 mcg/D5W 250 mLs at 11 mLs/hr).

-Fresh frozen plasma 2-4 units IV.

BACTERIAL CHOLANGITIS & BILIARY SEPSIS

History and Physical: Fever and chills, abdominal pain, and jaundice (Charcot's triad). findings include; icterus, hepatomegaly, ascites, and focal or diffuse abdominal tenderness.

Labs: CBC, SMA 12, LDH, amylase, lipase, blood C&S x 3. UA, PT/PTT.

Extras: CXR, ECG, RUQ & liver ultrasound, HIDA, acute abdomen series. GI & surgery consults.

Treatment:

-Mezlocillin, Azlocillin or Piperacillin 3 gm IV q4-6h **AND**
Metronidazole 500 mg (7.5 mg/kg) IV q6h **OR**

-Cefoxitin (Mefoxin) 1-2 gm IV q6-8h (with gentamicin) **OR**

-Ticarcillin/clavulanate (Timentin) 3.1 g IV q4-6h **OR**

-Ampicillin 1-2 gm IV q4-6h. **AND**
Gentamicin 100 mg (1.5-2 mg/kg), then 80 mg IV q8h (3-5 mg/kg/d) **AND**
Metronidazole 500 mg (7.5 mg/kg) IV q6h.

ACUTE PANCREATITIS

History and Physical: Abdominal pain usually localized to the epigastrium with radiation to the back or flank. Nausea and vomiting with a history of ethanol abuse, biliary disease, or abdominal surgery. Exam reveals fever, tachycardia, epigastric tenderness with guarding, hypotension, tachypnea, obtundation, and jaundice.

Labs: CBC, platelets, SMA 7 & 12, ionized & total calcium; triglycerides, amylase, lipase, LDH, SGOT, ABG, blood C&S x 3, coagulation panel, HEPATITIS B SURFACE ANTIGEN, PT/PTT, type & hold PRBC, FFP. Pancreatic isoamylase. UA.

Upright abdomen, CXR for tube placement, ECG, ultrasound, CT, 10-18 F NG tube at low constant suction (if obstruction). Foley to closed drainage.

Prognosis: Ranson's Criteria:

  At Admission:

    Age > 55

    WBC > 16,000/mm3

    Blood glucose > 200 mg/dL

    Serum LDH > 350 IU/l

    Serum SGOT > 250 u/dL

  During initial 48 hours:

    Hct fall > 10%

    BUN increases > 5 mg/dL

    Serum Calcium < 8 mg/dL

    Arterial p02 < 60 mm Hg

    Base deficit > 4 mEq/l

    Fluid sequestration > 61

Treatment:

1. IV fluid replacement for hypotension, tachycardia, decreased urine output. If severe, consider invasive monitoring.

2. Provide electrolyte replacement for hypokalemia, hypocalcemia, hypomagnesemia. Discontinue medications known to cause pancreatitis.

3. **H2 Blockers:**

    -Ranitidine (Zantac) 6.25-12.5 mg/h (0.2-0.4 mg/kg/h)(150- 300 mg in 500 mL D5W at 21 mL/h) IV or 50 mg IV q6-8h **OR**

    -Cimetidine (Tagamet) 37.5-50 mg/h IV or 300 mg IV q6-8h **OR**

    -Famotidine (Pepcid) 20 mg IV q12h.

4. **Volume Replacement:**

    -Albumin 25 gm IV (100 mL of 25% solution) or 250 mL 5% sln **OR**

    -Hetastarch (Hespan) 500-1000 mL over 30-60 min; max 1500 cc/d.

5. **Antibiotics:**

    -Cefoxitin (Mefoxin) 1-2 gm IV q6-8h **OR**

    -Ofloxacin (Oflox) or ciprofloxacin (Cipro) 400 mg IV q12h.

6. **Analgesia:** Meperidine 50-100 mg IM q3-4h prn pain.

7. **Total Parenteral Nutrition:** Required if malnutrition or inability to tolerate orals for >3-5 days. Lipids infusions may worsen pancreatitis; need to follow triglyceride levels.

8. **Indications for Surgical Intervention:** Uncertain diagnosis, deteriorating condition, biliary pancreatitis, and infected pancreatic necrosis and/or pancreatic abscess.

HEPATIC ENCEPHALOPATHY

History and Physical: Lethargy, confusion, stupor, and coma. Physical exam may reveal hepatosplenomegaly, ascites, jaundice, spider angiomas, gynecomastia, and testicular atrophy.

Labs: Ammonia, CBC, platelets, SMA 12, Mg, Cal, SGOT, SGPT, SGGT, LDH, alkaline phosphatase, protein, albumin, bilirubin, PT/PTT, ABG, hepatitis panel. UA. CXR, ECG, urine and blood drug screen. Blood and urine cultures.

General Measures: Avoid sedatives, diuretics, NSAIDS or hepatotoxic drugs. Turn patient q2h while awake, chart stools. Foley to closed drainage.

Treatment:

-Milk of magnesia 30 mg PO x 1 dose before starting lactulose (avoid if inadequate renal function.)

-Lactulose 30-45 mL PO q1h x 3 doses, then 15-45 mL PO bid-qid titrate to produce 2 soft stools/d. **OR**

-Lactulose enema 300 mL in 700 mL of tap water bid-qid **OR**

-Neomycin 0.5-1.0 gm PO/NG q4-6h (4-12 g/d).

Nutrition and Other Measures:

-Ranitidine (Zantac) 50 mg IV q6-8h or 150 mg PO bid **OR**

-Cimetidine (Tagamet) 37.5-50 mg/h IV or 300 mg IV q6-8h or 300 mg PO tid-qid **OR**

-Famotidine (Pepcid) 20 mg IV/PO q12h

-Vitamin K 10 mg SQ qd x 3d.

-Multivitamin PO qAM or 1 ampule IV qAM.

-Folic acid 1 mg PO/IV qd.

-Thiamine 100 mg PO/IV qd.

REFERENCES

Eastwood GL. In: Rippe JM; Irwin RS; Alpert JS; Fink MP. Intensive care medicine. 2nd ed. boston; Little, Brown and Company, 1991; 901-917.
Peterson WL; Barnett CC; Smith HJ; et.al: Routine early endoscopy in upper-gastrointestinal-tract bleeding. N Engl J Med 304:925, 1981.
Keller FS; Rosch J: Value of angiography in diagnosis and therapy of acute upper gastrointestinal hemorrhage. Dig Dis Sci 26:78s, 1981.
Som P; Oster ZH; Atkins HL; et.al.: Detection of gastrointestinal blood loss with 99mTc-labeled, heat-treated red blood cells. Radiology 138:207, 1981.
Dawson J; Cockel R: Ranitidine in acute upper gastrointestinal hemorrhage. Be Med J 285:476, 1982.
Groll A; Simon JB; Wigle RD; et.al.: Cimetidine prophylaxis for gastrointestinal bleeding in an intensive care unit. Gut 27:135, 1986.
Kadakia SC: Biliary tract emergencies. Acute cholocystitis, acute cholangitis, and acute pancreatitis. Medical Clinics of North America 77:1015, 1993.
Kuvshinoff BW; McFadden DW. In: Rippe JM; Irwin RS; Alpert JS; Fink MP. Intensive care medicine. 2nd ed. Boston: Little, Brown and Company, 1991; 1326-1334.
Sung JJY, etal: Octreotide infusion or emergency sclerotherapy for variceal hemorrhage. Lancet 1993; 342: 637-41.

Adams L; Soulen MC. TIPS: a new alternative for the variceal bleeder. Am J Crit Care 2:196, 1993.

Smith SL; Ciferni M. Liver transplantation for acute hepatic failure: a review of clinical experience and and management. Am J Crit Care 2:137, 1993.

Bucci L; Palmieri GC. Double-blind, double-dummy comparison between treatment with rifaximin and lactulose in patients with medium to severe degree hepatic encephalopathy. Current Medical Research and Opinion 13:109, 1993.

Davenport A; Will EJ; Davison AM. Effect of renal replacement therapy on patients with combined acute renal and fulminant hepatic failure. Kidney International. Supplement 41:S245, 1993.

Fingerote RJ; Bain VG. Fulminant hepatic failure. American J of Gastroenterlogy 88:1000, 1993.

TOXICOLOGY

By Humphrey Wong, MD

POISONING AND DRUG OVERDOSE

Management of Poisoning and Drug Overdose:

1. Stabilize vital signs; maintain airway, breathing and circulation.
2. Consider intubation if patient has depressed mental status and is at risk for aspiration or respiratory failure.
3. Establish IV access and administer oxygen.
4. Evaluate for ingestion of multiple drugs. Determine the type and quantity of substances ingested.
5. Prevent further absorption of toxin; administer antidote if available; enhance elimination of toxin.
6. Reassess response to therapy, and continue supportive care.
7. Contact regional poison control center for guidance and updated management.

General Management of Altered Mental Status:

1. Draw blood for baseline labs (see below):
2. D50W 50 mLs IV push, followed by Naloxone (Narcan) 2 mg IV, followed by Thiamine 100 mg IV.
3. Consider Flumazenil (Romazicon) 0.2 mg IV up to 3 - 5 mg IV if no response. Excessive flumazenil may precipitate seizures. Flumazenil reverses CNS depression, but not respiratory depression.
4. If no improvement, evaluate for other causes of altered mental status.

Labs:

-CBC, SMA-6, glucose, liver function tests, INR/PTT; CPK, serum and urine toxicology screen; arterial blood gas, urinalysis; EKG, CXR.
-Be aware of the drugs included and not included in your hospital's screen panel. A particular drug may need to be specifically assayed for if suspected, eg. lithium.

Gastrointestinal Decontamination:

Gastric Lavage:

1. Contraindications: Suspected acid, alkali, hydrocarbon, or sharp object ingestion.
2. Consider intubation for airway protection if depressed mental status.
3. Place the patient in Trendelenburg's position and left lateral decubitus. Insert a large bore (32-40) french Ewald oral gastric tube. A smaller NG tube may be used but may be less effective in retrieving large particles.
4. After tube placement has been confirmed by auscultation, aspirate stomach contents and lavage with 200 cc aliquots of saline or water until clear up to 2 L.

5. Send the first 100 cc for toxicology analysis.

Activated Charcoal (AC):

A. Not effective for alcohols, aliphatic hydrocarbons, caustics, cyanide, elemental metals (boric acid, iron, lithium, lead), or pesticides.

B. Oral dose is 1 g/kg or 10:1 ratio of charcoal to amount of drug ingested. May repeat dose of 0.5-1.0 g/kg q4h if massive ingestion, sustained release products, cyclic antidepressants, carbamazepine, digoxin, phenobarbital, phenytoin, valproate, salicylate, doxepin, theophylline, and quinine.

C. Give oral cathartic with charcoal (70% sorbitol). Contraindicated in infants and patients with ileus. Use magnesium with caution in renal insufficiency.

Whole Bowel Irrigation (WBI):

A. Can prevent further absorption in cases of massive ingestion, delayed presentation, or in overdoses of enteric coated or sustained release pills.

B. May be useful in eliminating objects, such as batteries, or ingested packets of drugs.

C. Administer GoLytely, or Colyte orally at 1.6 - 2.0 l/hour until fecal effluent is clear. Contraindicated in patients with ileus.

Hemodialysis: Indications: phenobarbital, theophylline, chloral hydrate, salicylate, ethanol, lithium, ethylene glycol, isopropyl alcohol, procainamide, and methanol, severe metabolic acidosis.

Hemoperfusion (charcoal or resin):

-May be more effective than hemodialysis **except** for bromides, heavy metals, lithium, and ethylene glycol.

-Effective for chloramphenicol, disopyramide, phenytoin, ethchlorvynol, glutethimide, meprobamate, methaqualone, barbiturates, theophylline.

Forced Alkaline Diuresis:

-Enhances renal excretion of the ionized drug.

-Weak acids are more effectively removed in an alkaline pH.

-Consider use for salicylates, phenobarbital, sulfonamides.

-Use 3 amps $NaHCO_3$ in 1 L D5W. Keep urine pH between 7.5-8.5, and maintain urine output at 2-4 cc/kg/hour

-Watch for CHF, electrolyte imbalances, and follow arterial blood gases.

TOXICOLOGIC SYNDROMES

Characteristics of Common Toxicologic Syndromes:

A. **Cholinergic (muscarinic) Poisoning:** Salivation, defecation, lacrimation, emesis, urination, miosis.

B. **Anticholinergic Poisoning:** Dry skin, flushing, fever, urinary retention, mydriasis, thirst, delirium, conduction delays, tachycardia, ileus.

C. **Sympathomimetic Poisoning:** Agitation, hypertension, seizure, tachycardia, mydriasis, vasoconstriction.

D. **Narcotic Poisoning:** Lethargy, hypotension, hypoventilation, miosis, coma, ileus.

E. **Withdrawal Syndrome:** diarrhea, lacrimation, mydriasis, cramps, tachycardia, hallucination.

F. **Common Causes of Toxic Seizures:** Amoxapine, anticholinergics, camphor, carbon monoxide, cocaine, ergotamine, isoniazid, lead, lindane, lithium, LSD, parathion, phencyclidine, phenothiazines, propoxyphene HCL, propranolol, strychnine, theophylline, tricyclic antidepressants.

G. **Common Causes of Toxic Cardiac Arrhythmias:** Arsenic, beta-blockers, chloral hydrate, chloroquine, clonidine, calcium channel blockers, cocaine, cyanide, carbon monoxide, digitalis, ethanol, phenol, phenothiazine, physostigmine, quinine, succinylcholine, tricyclics.

MANAGEMENT OF SPECIFIC OVERDOSES

ACETAMINOPHEN OVERDOSE

General Information:

-Acute lethal dose = 13 - 25 g.

-Acetaminophen is partly metabolized to N-acetyl-p-benzoquinonimine which is conjugated by glutathione, which can be depleted in overdoses, leading to centrilobular necrosis.

Signs and Symptoms:

-Liver failure occurs 3 days after ingestion if untreated; presents with right upper quadrant pain, elevated liver function tests, coagulopathy, hypoglycemia, renal failure, and encephalopathy.

Treatment:

1. **Gastrointestinal Decontamination:** Gastric lavage followed by activated charcoal. Remove residual charcoal with saline lavage prior to giving N-Acetyl-Cysteine (NAC).

2. Check 4 hour, post ingestion acetaminophen level. Use nomogram to determine if treatment is necessary (see next page). Start treatment if level is above the nontoxic range or if the level is potentially toxic but the time of ingestion is unknown.

3. Therapy must start no later than 8-12 hours after ingestion. Treatment after 16-24 hours is significantly less effective.

4. Oral NAC: NAC 140 mg/kg PO followed by 70 mg/kg PO q4h x 17 doses (total 1330 mg/kg over 72 h). Repeat loading dose x 1 if emesis occurs.

5. If oral route is not possible, the following protocol is available (but not FDA approved): NAC 150 mg/kg in 200 mL D5W IV over 15 min, followed by 50 mg/kg in 500 mL D5W IV over 4h, followed by 100 mg/kg in 1000 mL D5W IV over next 16 hours. Filter solution through 0.22 micron filter prior to administration. Complete all PO/NG/IV doses even after acetaminophen level falls below critical value.

6. Hemodialysis and hemoperfusion are somewhat effective, but should not take the place of NAC treatment.

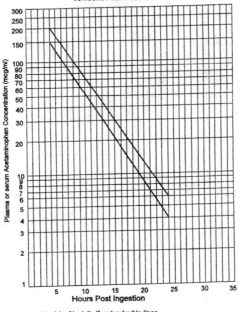

INTERPRETATION OF ACTAMINOPHEN LEVEL
VS HOURS POST INGESTION

No risk of toxicity if under double lines
Probable risk if above top line
Possible risk if between double lines
Outcome is best if treatment is initiated within 12 hours of
ingestion

CALCIUM CHANNEL BLOCKER OVERDOSE

Signs and Symptoms:
-Hypotension, bradycardia, AV node conduction block, heart failure, depressed mental status, hyperglycemia, nausea, vomiting.

Treatment:
1. Gastrointestinal decontamination with gastric lavage. Fluid resuscitation with NS or lactated Ringer's.
2. Calcium chloride 1-2 g IV over 5-20 minutes.
3. Atropine 1-2 mg IV for bradycardia.
4. Epinephrine or dopamine infusion for hypotension.
5. Transvenous pacing
6. If above fails, consider:
   -Dobutamine 5-15 mcg/kg/min IV infusion.
   -Isoproterenol 2-10 mcg/min IV infusion.
   -Milrinone 50 mcg/kg IV over 10 min, then 0.375-0.75 mcg/kg/min IV infusion.
   -Glucagon 5-10 mg IV bolus, then 2-5 mg/h IV infusion.
   -Hemodialysis is not useful.

CAUSTIC INGESTION

Signs and Symptoms:
-Burns and inflammation of the oropharynx; retrosternal or abdominal pain; hematemesis, dysphagia.
-Acids may present with immediate pain; main site of injury is the gastric outlet.
-Bases may present with delayed pain; main site of injury is the esophagus.

Treatment: Acid and base solutions are treated similarly.
1. Evaluate for airway obstruction.
2. Fluid resuscitation for hypovolemia.
3. Attempt to rinse out oral cavity. Dilution of caustic with water should be considered. Do not attempt gastric lavage, emesis, charcoal, or neutralization.
4. Esophagogastroduodenoscopy or surgery may be indicated in 48 hours if injury is severe.
5. Rule out gastric perforation by chest and upright abdomen X-ray (ie pneumothorax, pneumomediastinum, pleural effusion, or abdominal free air).

COCAINE OVERDOSE

General Information:

A. Can be abused intravenously, smoked, ingested, or inhaled nasally. The effect of oral cocaine is equivalent to the intranasal route.

B. Street cocaine comes in unreliable concentrations, and often is cut with other substances including amphetamines, LSD, PCP, heroin, strychnine, lidocaine, talc, and quinine.

C. One-third of fatalities occur within 1 hour, with another third occurring 6 to 24 h later.

D. Be aware of "body packers" who transport cocaine by swallowing well wrapped packets, and "body stuffers" who hastily swallow packets of cocaine to avoid arrest.

Signs and Symptoms:

A. **CNS:** Sympathetic stimulation, agitation, seizures, tremor, headache, subarachnoid hemorrhage, cerebral vascular accident, psychosis, hallucinations, fever, mydriasis, formication (sensation of insects crawling on skin).

B. **Cardiovascular:** Atrial and ventricular arrhythmias, myocardial infarction; hypertension, hypotension, myocarditis, aortic rupture, cardiomyopathy.

C. **Pulmonary:** Noncardiogenic pulmonary edema; pneumomediastinum, alveolar hemorrhage; hypersensitivity pneumonitis, bronchiolitis obliterans.

D. **Other:** Rhabdomyolysis, mesenteric ischemia, hepatitis.

Treatment:

1. Supportive care. No antidote is available.

2. GI Decontamination, including repeated activated charcoal, whole bowel irrigation, and endoscopic evaluation if oral or packet ingestion suspected.

3. Treat hyperadrenergic symptoms with benzodiazepines such as diazepam.

Seizures:

1. Treat with diazepam, phenytoin, or phenobarbital.

2. Evaluate for other possible causes such as subarachnoid hemorrhage, hypoxemia, and hypoglycemia.

Arrhythmias:

1. Treat hyper-adrenergic state and supraventricular tachycardia with diazepam and propranolol.

2. Treat ventricular arrhythmias with lidocaine or bretylium. Propranolol may be required.

Hypertension:

1. Use diazepam first for tachycardia and hypertension.

2. If no response, use labetalol for alpha and beta blocking effects.

3. If hypertension remains severe, consider sodium nitroprusside and esmolol drips.

Myocardial Ischemia and Infarction:

1. Treat with thrombolysis, heparin, aspirin, beta-blockers as indicated.
2. Control hypertension and consider possibility of CNS bleed before using thrombolytic therapy if indicated.

CYANIDE INGESTION

<u>General Information:</u> One of the most rapidly lethal poisons; Found in industrial settings involving metallurgy, plastics, and in fires involving synthetic fibers and plastics. Toxicity may occur with prolonged use of sodium nitroprusside drips.

Mechanism: Cyanide has high affinity to Fe^{+3} leading to inhibition of the cytochrome system, thus blocking aerobic respiration, and leading to death.

Toxicity: 50 mg Cyanide orally is fatal.

<u>Signs and Symptoms:</u>

1. **Excitement Phase:** Anxiety, dyspnea, confusion, tachycardia.
2. **Depression Phase:** Visual change, seizure, bradycardia, hypotension, hypoventilation.
3. **Adynamic Phase:** Coma, hypotonia and areflexia, hemodynamic collapse; severe lactic acidosis with high mixed venous oxygen saturation.

<u>Treatment:</u>

1. Intubation, 100% oxygen, or hyperbaric oxygen.
2. Cardiopulmonary resuscitation and GI decontamination.
3. Amyl nitrate Perles: Inhale 1 Perle (0.2 mL) over 30 seconds every minute until IV access available.
4. Sodium nitrate: 10 mL of 3 % solution (300 mg) IV over 3 minutes.
5. Sodium Thiosulfate: 50 mL of 25% solution (12,500 mg) IV over 10 minutes.
6. Follow methemoglobin levels.

CYCLIC ANTIDEPRESSANT OVERDOSE

General Information:
- Has large volume of distribution (15-40 L/kg), high lipid solubility, high protein binding. Prolonged body clearance rates, and ineffective removal by forced diuresis, hemodialysis, and hemoperfusion.
- Expect possibly delayed absorption due to decreased GI motility from anticholinergic effects.

Signs and Symptoms:
CNS: Lethargy, coma, hallucinations, seizures, myoclonic jerks.

Anticholinergic crises: Blurred vision, dilated pupils, urinary retention, dry mouth, ileus, hyperthermia.

Cardiac: Hypotension, ventricular tachyarrhythmias, heart block.

EKG: Sinus tachycardia, right bundle branch block, right axis deviation, increased PR and QT interval, QRS > 100 msec, or right axis deviation. Prolongation of the QRS width is a more reliable predictor of CNS and cardiac toxicity than the TCA level.

Treatment:
1. **Gastrointestinal Decontamination and Systemic Drug Removal:**

   Magnesium citrate 300 mLs via nasogastric tube x 1 dose.

   Activated charcoal premixed with sorbitol 50 gms via nasogastric tube q4-6h around-the-clock until TCA level decreases to therapeutic range. Maintain the head-of-bed at a 30-45 degree angle to prevent aspiration.

2. **Cardiac Toxicity:**

   Alkalinization is a cardioprotective measure and it has no influence on drug elimination. Treatment goal is to achieve an arterial pH of 7.50-7.55.

   If mechanical ventilation is necessary, hyperventilate to maintain desired pH.

   Administer sodium bicarbonate 50-100 mEq (1-2 amps or 1-2 mEq/kg) IV over 5-10 min. Followed by infusion of sodium bicarbonate 2 amps in 1 liter of D5W at 100-150 cc/h. Adjust IV rate to maintain desired pH.

3. **Seizures:**

   Lorazepam or diazepam IV followed by phenytoin (see page 125)

   Consider physostigmine 1-2 mg slow IV over 3-4 min if seizures continue.

DIGOXIN OVERDOSE

General Information:
-Therapeutic window is 0.8-2.0 ng/mL. Serum digoxin levels are most accurate if drawn 4 hours after an IV dose and 6 hours after a PO dose.
-Drug-drug interactions that increase digoxin levels include verapamil, quinidine, amiodarone, flecainide, erythromycin, and tetracycline.
-Hypokalemia, hypomagnesemia and hypercalcemia enhance digoxin toxicity.

Signs and Symptoms:
CNS: Confusion, lethargy; yellow-green visual halo.

Cardiac: Any dysrhythmia can be seen including atrial fibrillation and flutter, VT; VF, bidirectional VT variable AV block, AV dissociation; sinus bradycardia, junctional tachycardia, PVC's.

GI: Nausea, vomiting

Metabolic: Hyperkalemia is common but may be normal or low in patients on diuretics.

Treatment:
1. **Gastrointestinal Decontamination:** Bradycardia or asystole may result from vagal stimulation during gastric lavage; repeated doses of activated charcoal are effective; hemodialysis is ineffective.
2. Treat bradycardia with atropine, isoproterenol, and cardiac pacing.
3. Treat ventricular arrhythmias with lidocaine or phenytoin. Avoid procainamide and quinidine as they may be proarrhythmic and slow AV conduction.
4. Electrical DC cardioversion may be dangerous in severe toxicity, and should be used judiciously and at low energy settings.
5. Correct hypomagnesemia and hypokalemia.

Digibind (Digoxin - specific Fab antibody fragment):
-Indication: life threatening arrhythmias refractory to conventional therapy.
-Dosage of Digoxin immune Fab

$$(\text{number of 40 mg vials}) = \frac{\text{Digoxin level (ng/mL) x body weight (kg)}}{100}$$

-Dissolve the digoxin immune Fab in 100-150 mLs of NS and infuse IV over 15-30 minutes. Use a 0.22 micron in-line filter during infusion.
-Watch for hypokalemia, heart failure, anaphylaxis. Complex is renally excreted; after administration, serum digoxin level may be high and inaccurate because both free and bound digoxin is measured with certain assays.

ETHANOL OVERDOSE

General Information:
-Evaluate for coingestion of other drugs, occult trauma, Wernicke's encephalopathy, alcoholic ketoacidosis, infections, dehydration, GI bleed, hypoglycemia, electrolyte derangement (eg. Mg , K, phosphate).

Toxicity:
-Lethal dose: 5-8 g/kg
-Lethal blood level: 350-500 mg/dL (variably dependent on tolerance)

Time of Onset of Alcohol Related Illness:
-Seizures: 6-48 hours
-Withdrawal: 6-72 hours
-Delirium tremens: 4-7 days (carries 9-15% mortality)

Signs and Symptoms: Seizures, Withdrawal, Delirium.

Treatment:
1. Provide supportive care.
2. Treat seizures with diazepam 5-10 mg IV push.
3. Withdrawal: Chlordiazepoxide (Librium) 50-100 mg IV q6h around-the-clock x 48-72 hours.
4. Magnesium sulfate 2 gms, multivitamins 10 mLs, thiamine 100 mg, folic acid 1 mg in 1 liter of IV fluids qd.

ETHYLENE GLYCOL INGESTION

General Information: Found in antifreeze, detergents, and polishes.

Toxicity: Half-life 3-5 hours; increases to 17 h if coingested with alcohol; minimal lethal dose 1.0-1.5 cc/kg; lethal blood level 200 mg/dL

Signs and Symptoms:
-Anion gap metabolic acidosis and severe osmolar gap
-CNS depression; cranial nerve dysfunction (facial and vestibulocochlear palsies)
-GI symptoms such as flank pain; oxalate crystals in urine sediment; hypocalcemia (due to calcium oxalate formation); tetany, seizures, and prolonged QT may occur.

Treatment:
1. 10 % Ethanol (in D5W) as 7.5 cc/kg IV load, then 1.4 cc/kg/h IV drip to keep blood alcohol level between 100-150 mg/dL and to keep serum ethylene glycol level < 10 mg/dL.
2. Pyridoxine 100 mg IV qid x 2 days and thiamine 100 mg IV qid x 2 days; may increase metabolism of glyoxylate.

3.   If definitive therapy is delayed, give 3-4 ounces of whiskey (or equivalent) orally.
4.   **Hemodialysis:**
     -Indications: Severe acidosis, crystalluria, serum ethylene glycol level > 50 mg/dL; keep glycol level <10 mg/dL.

ISOPROPYL ALCOHOL INGESTION

General Information: Found in rubbing alcohol, solvents, and antifreeze.

Toxicity: Lethal dose: 3-4 g/kg
   -Lethal blood level : 400 mg/dL
   -Half life = 3 hours

Metabolism: Isopropyl alcohol is metabolized to acetone

Signs and Symptoms:
   -Anion gap metabolic acidosis with high serum ketone level; mild osmol gap; mildly elevated glucose.
   -CNS depression, headache, nystagmus; cardiovascular depression; abdominal pain and vomiting; pulmonary edema.

Treatment:
1.   Provide supportive care. No antidote available; ethanol is not indicated.
2.   **Hemodialysis:**   Indications: refractory hypotension, coma state, potentially lethal blood levels.

METHANOL INGESTION

General Information: Found in antifreeze, Sterno, cleaners, paints.

Toxicity:
   -10 cc causes blindness
   -Minimal lethal dose = 1-5 g/kg
   -Lethal blood level = 80 mg/dL
   -Symptomatic in 40 min to 72 h.

Signs and Symptoms:
   -Severe osmol and anion gap metabolic acidosis.
   -Visual changes due to optic nerve toxicity, leading to blindness.
   -Nausea, vomiting, abdominal pain, pancreatitis; altered mental status.

Treatment:
1.   Infuse 10% ethanol (in D5W) as 7.5 cc/kg load then 1.4 cc/kg/h drip to keep blood alcohol level between 100-150 mg/dL. Continue therapy

until methanol level is below 20 - 25 mg/dL. Consider continuing therapy for a few days because ethanol increases methanol half life to 24-30h.

2. Give folate 50 mg IV q4h to enhance formic acid metabolism.

3. If definitive therapy is delayed, give 3-4 ounces of whiskey (or equivalent) orally.

4. Correct acidosis and electrolyte imbalances.

5. **Hemodialysis:**

-Indications: peak methanol level > 50 mg/dL; formic acid level > 20 mg/dL; severe metabolic acidosis; acute renal failure; any visual compromise.

IRON OVERDOSE

General Information: $FeSO_4$ is 20% elemental iron and ferrous gluconate contains 12%.

Toxicity:

-Nontoxic: <10-20 mg/kg (0-100 mcg/dL)

-Toxic: > 20 mg/kg (350-1000 mcg/dL)

-Lethal: >180-300 mg/kg (>1000 mcg/dL)

-Toxicity is due to of free radicals and tissue damage to the GI mucosa, liver, kidney, heart and lungs. Cause of death is usually shock and liver failure.

Metabolism:

Signs and Symptoms:

Two Hours After Ingestion:

-Severe hemorrhagic gastritis; vomiting, diarrhea, lethargy, tachycardia, hypotension.

Twelve Hours After Ingestion:

-Improvement and stabilization.

12-48 Hours After Ingestion:

-GI bleeding, coma, seizures, pulmonary edema, circulatory collapse; hepatic and renal failure; coagulopathy, hypoglycemia, severe metabolic acidosis.

4-6 Weeks After Ingestion:

-Gastric scarring and recovery.

Treatment:

1. Administer deferoxamine antidote. 100 mg of deferoxamine binds 9 mg of free elemental iron.

2. Deferoxamine Dosage:

IM 40-90 mg/kg; max 2 gm per injection or 6 gms per day.

IV 15 mg/kg/h; max 6 gms per day.

3. Treat until 24 hours after vin rose colored urine clears. Serum iron levels during chelation are not accurate.
4. **Gastrointestinal Decontamination:**
    -Charcoal is not effective in absorbing elemental iron. Evaluate x-rays for remaining iron tablets. Consider white bowel lavage if iron pills are past the stomach and cannot be removed by lavage, see page 102.
5. **Hemodialysis:** Consider for severe toxicity.

LITHIUM OVERDOSE

General Information:
-Has a narrow therapeutic window of 0.8-1.2 mEq/l.
-Drug-drug interactions will increase lithium levels: NSAID's: (indomethacin, ibuprofen, piroxicam); phenothiazines, thiazides; Aldactone.

Toxicity:
1.5-3.0 mEq/l = moderate toxicity
3.0-4.0 mEq/l = severe toxicity
-Toxicity in chronic lithium users occurs at much lower serum levels than with acute ingestions.

Signs and Symptoms:
-Seizure, encephalopathy, hyperreflexia, tremor, nausea, vomiting, diarrhea, hypotension; nephrogenic diabetes insipidus, hypothyroidism. Conduction block and dysrhythmias are rare, but reversible T wave depression may occur.

Treatment:
-Correct hyponatremia; hyponatremia increases proximal renal tubule reabsorption of lithium
-Follow lithium levels until < 1.0 mEq/l and watch for rebound as levels may increase from intracellular stores.

Forced Solute Diuresis:
-Hydrate with normal saline infusion to maintain urine output at 2-4 cc/kg/hr; use furosemide (Lasix) 40-80 mg IV doses as needed if euvolemic and hyponatremia is absent.

GI Decontamination:
-Administer gastric lavage.
-Activated charcoal is ineffective. Consider whole bowel irrigation.

Indications for Hemodialysis: Level >4 mEq/l; chronic ingestion with symptoms; CNS or cardiovascular impairment with level of 2.5-4.0 mEq/l.

OPIATE OVERDOSE

General Information:
-Opiates include morphine, heroin, codeine, fentanyl, hydromorphone, methadone, propoxyphene, diphenoxylate, methadone.

-The concentration and purity of elicit opiate is highly variable, leading to increased incidence of toxicity. Adulterates includes: mannitol, talc, quinine, strychnine, lidocaine, amphetamines, barbiturates, PCP.

-Designer drugs such as alpha-methyl-fentanyl (China White) can be up to 3000 times as potent as heroin causing accidental overdoses.

Signs and Symptoms:
-Miosis (except mydriasis for diphenoxylate or meperidine); respiratory depression; CNS depression.

-Pulmonary edema, arteritis, thrombosis, septic emboli, pneumonia, abscess.

-Seizures seen with meperidine, propoxyphene, pentazocine, fentanyl.

-Hypotension; rhabdomyolysis, acute renal failure.

Treatment:
1. Provide supportive care.
2. Naloxone (Narcan) 0.4-2.0 mg IV/ET q2min, up to 10 mg; **OR** 0.005 mg/kg IVP followed by 0.0025 mg/kg/h IV infusion. Very high doses may be needed for pentazocine, diphenoxylate, methadone, and propoxyphene ingestion.
3. Watch for withdrawal symptoms.
4. Evaluate for coingestions of other drugs.

SALICYLATE OVERDOSE

Toxicity:
-150-300 mg/kg - mild toxicity

-300-500 mg/kg - moderate toxicity

- > 500 mg/kg - severe toxicity

-Chronic use can cause toxicity at much lower levels (ie. 25 mg/dL) than occurs with acute use.

Signs and Symptoms:
Acid/Base Abnormalities: Patients present initially with a respiratory alkalosis due to central hyperventilation; later an anion gap metabolic acidosis occurs.

CNS: Tinnitus, lethargy, irritability, seizures, coma, cerebral edema.

GI: Nausea, vomiting, liver failure, GI bleeding.

Cardiac: Hypotension, sinus tachycardia, AV block, wide complex tachycardia

Pulmonary: Non-cardiogenic pulmonary edema, adult respiratory distress syndrome.

Other: Renal failure; coagulopathy due to decreased factor VII; hyperthermia due to uncoupled oxidative phosphorylation.

Treatment:

1. Provide supportive care and GI decontamination. Consider possibility of concretion or drug bezoar formation, or ingestion of enteric coated preparations which may lead to delayed toxicity.
2. Consider multiple dose activated charcoal, and whole bowel irrigation, and follow serial salicylate levels.
3. Treat hypotension and dehydration vigorously with fluids, and correct electrolytes, especially potassium. Maintain urine output at 200 cc/h or more.
4. Correct metabolic acidosis with bicarbonate 50-100 mEq (1-2 amps) IVP.
5. Alkalinize urine with IV bicarbonate infusion (2-3 amps in 1 liter of D5W at 150-200 mL/h), keeping the urine pH at 7.5-8.5 (significantly increases renal clearance).

Hemodialysis or charcoal hemoperfusion:

-Indications: Seizures, cardiac or renal failure, intractable acidosis, acute salicylate level > 120 mg/dL or chronic level > 50 mg/dL (therapeutic level 15-25 mg/dL).

-Hemoperfusion is effective in clearance of salicylate, but less effective at correcting electrolyte and acid-base imbalances.

SEDATIVE-HYPNOTIC OVERDOSE

General Information:

-Sedative hypnotics include antihistamines, meprobamate, barbiturates, methaqualone, benzodiazepines, chloral hydrate, glutethimide.

-Drugs in barbiturate class are highly subject to abuse, either alone, or usually in combination with heroin. Effects are worsened with alcohol.

Signs and Symptoms:

-Sedation to coma, hypotension, respiratory depression.

-Anticholinergic symptoms with glutethimide, and antihistamines.

-Seizures may occur with methaqualone, glutethimide, and ethchlorvynol.

-Arrhythmias may occur with chloral hydrate.

Treatment:

1. Provide supportive care and GI decontamination. Bezoars may form with meprobamate.

2. Support blood pressure with volume and pressor agents.
3. Forced alkaline diuresis in cases of barbiturate, and meprobamate ingestion.
4. Consider hemoperfusion or hemodialysis for persistent hemodynamic instability refractory to therapy.
5. Watch for signs of withdrawal.

Flumazenil (Romazicon) for benzodiazepine ingestions:

-0.2 mg IV initially, then 0.5 mg IV q 30 seconds up to 3 to 5 mg IV total; Is more effective for reversal of sedation than for reversal of hypoventilation. Flumazenil can precipitate seizures if given in excess of the amount required to reverse benzodiazepine effects. Contraindicated in concurrent cyclic antidepressant overdose.

THEOPHYLLINE TOXICITY

General Information:

-Drug interactions can increase serum levels: Quinolone and macrolide antibiotics, propranolol, cimetidine, and oral contraceptives.
-Liver disease or heart failure will decrease clearance; PEEP may decrease cardiac output and thus may decrease drug clearance.

Toxicity:

-Acute toxicity: Serum levels;

20-40 mg/dL - mild

40-70 mg/dL - moderate

70 + mg/dL - life threatening

-Acute and chronic toxicity differ in that chronic users can suffer toxicity at lower serum levels; there is less correlation between serum levels and symptoms; seizures and arrhythmias can occur at therapeutic or mildly supratherapeutic levels.

Signs and Symptoms:

CNS: Hyperventilation, agitation, and tonic-clonic seizures.

Cardiac: Sinus tachycardia, multi-focal atrial tachycardia, supraventricular tachycardia, VT, VF, PVC's, hypotension or hypertension.

GI: Vomiting, diarrhea, hematemesis.

Musculoskeletal: Tremor, myoclonic jerks

Metabolic: Decreased K, Mg, phosphate, and increased glucose, calcium and lactate.

Treatment:

1. **GI Decontamination and Systemic Drug Removal:**

-Activated charcoal premixed with sorbitol, 50 gms PO or via nasogastric tube q4-6h around-the-clock until theophylline level <20 mcg/mL. Maintain head-of-bed at 30-45 degrees to prevent charcoal aspiration.

2. **Indications for Charcoal Hemoperfusion:** Coma, seizures, hemodynamic instability, theophylline level > 60 mcg/mL; watch attach for rebound in serum level after discontinuation of hemoperfusion.

3. **Seizures** may be refractory to standard therapy with diazepam, dilantin, and phenobarbital. Seizures indicate a poor prognosis and mortality of up to 50%.

4. **Treat Hypotension** with fluids.
    Norepinephrine 8-12 mcg/min IV infusion or
    Phenylephrine 0.04-1.8 mg/min IV infusion.

5. **Treat Arrhythmias:**
    -Lidocaine 1 mg/kg loading up to 3 mg/kg, then 1-4 mg/min continuous IV drip **OR**
    -Esmolol (Brevibloc) 500 mcg/kg/min loading dose, then 50-300 mcg/kg/min continuous IV drip.

CLINICAL TOXICOLOGIC CONDITIONS

Radiopaque Drugs: Chloral hydrate, phenothiazines, cocaine packets, tricyclic antidepressants, calcium, potassium, heavy metals, enteric coated tablets, iron, iodine.

Drugs That Form Concretions: Iron, barbiturates, meprobamate, ethchlorvynol, salicylates, lithium, glutethimide, sustained release theophylline.

Causes of Elevated Osmolar Gap: Ethanol, methanol, isopropanol , ethylene glycol, glycerol, acetone, mannitol, sorbitol, hyperproteinemia hyperlipidemia.

Causes of Anion Gap Acidosis: Salicylates, methanol, ethylene glycol, paraldehyde, toluene, iron, isoniazid, strychnine, ketoacidosis (diabetic, alcoholic, starvation), uremia, lactate.

Osmolar Gap = calculated osmolarity - measured osmolarity

Osmolality = $2 \times Na + \dfrac{glucose}{18} + \dfrac{BUN}{2.8} + \dfrac{ETOH}{4.6}$

Anion Gap = $Na - (Cl + HCO3)$

REFERENCES

Bernstein G, Jehle D, et al.: Failure of Gastric Emptying and Charcoal Administration in Fatal Sustained-Release Theophylline Overdose: Pharmacobezoar Formation. Annals of Emergency Medicine, 21:1388 , 1993

Doyon S, Roberts, Jr.: The Use of Glucagon in a Case of Calcium Channel Blocker Overdose. Annals of Emergency Medicine, 22:1229, 1993.

Ellenhorn MJ, Barceloux DG (eds.): Medical Toxicology, Elsevier Science Publishing, 1988

Hall JB, Schmidt GA, Wood LDH (eds):Principles of Critical Care, New York, McGraw-Hill, 1992.

Harchelroad F, Cottington E, Krenzelok, EP: Gastrointestinal Transit Times of a Charcoal/Sorbitol Slurry in Overdose Patients. Clinical Toxicology, 27:91, 1989.

Kelly RA, Smith TW: Recognition and Management of Digitalis Toxicity. The American Journal of Cardiology,69:108G, 1992

Markenson D, Greenberg MD: Cyclic Antidepressant Overdose: Mechanism to Management. Emergency Medicine, 25:49, 1993.

Prescott LF: Treatment of Severe Acetaminophen Poisoning with Intravenous Acetylcysteine. Arch Intern Med. 1981; 141:386-9

Prescott LF, et al: Intravenous Acetylcysteine. Br Med J 1979; 2:1097-100

Rippe JM, Irwin RS, Alpert JS, Fink MP (eds): Intensive Care Medicine, 2nd ed. Boston, Little, Brown and Company, 1991.

Rosen, Peter (ed.): Emergency Medicine, Concepts and Clinical Practice, 3rd ed. Mosby Year Book, 1992

Smilkstein MJ, Bronstein AC, et al.: Acetaminophen Overdose: A 48-hour Intravenous N-Acetylcysteine Treatment Protocol. Annals of Emergency Medicine, 20:1058, 1991.

Spiller HA, Kreuzelok EP, Grand GA, et al.: A Prospective Evaluation of the Effect of Activated Charcoal before Oral N-Acetylcysteine in Acetaminophen Overdose. Annals of Emergency Medicine, 23:519-523, 1994.

Cooling DS. Theophylline Toxicity. Journal of Emergency Medicine, 11 (4):415-25, 1993.

Wolf LR, Spadafora MP, Otten EJ: Use of Amrinone and Glucagon in a Case of Calcium Channel Blocker Overdose. Annals of Emergency Medicine, 22:1225, 1993

Wolfe TR, Caravati EM, Rollins DE: Terminal 40-ms Frontal Plane QRS Axis as Marker for Tricyclic Antidepressant Overdose. Annals of Emergency Medicine, 18:348, 1989.

NEUROLOGY

By Jeffrey McGovern, M.D.

MANAGEMENT OF THE UNCONSCIOUS PATIENT

1. **Maintain Airway, Breathing, Circulation,** and administer oxygen.
2. **Obtain Labs:** CBC, electrolytes, creatinine, BUN, magnesium, calcium, glucose, toxicology screen, type and cross, liver function test, PT/PTT. Blood cultures, alcohol level.
3. **Administer Glucose,** 25 gm (50 mL of 50% dextrose IV push). Naloxone (Narcan) 0.4-2.0 mg IV/IM/ET.
4. **Consider measures to reduce elevated intracranial pressure (see page ?):**
5. **Control Seizures:**
   -Lorazepam (Ativan) 4-8 mg or diazepam (Valium) 5-10 mg IV push followed by dilantin.
6. **Nuchal Rigidity:** Lumbar puncture and panculture followed by antibiotic therapy for meningitis.
7. Evaluate pH, and correct acid/base disorders. Normalize temperature; consider administration of thiamine 100 mg IV push. Protect against bright light, and provide sedation for agitation.

ISCHEMIC STROKE

Presentation: Hemiparesis, seizure, delirium, syncope, dizziness/vertigo, coma.

Diagnosis: Complete neurologic exam; CT head (without contrast) to rule out intracranial hemorrhage; EKG; chest radiograph; complete chemistry screen, CBC, PT/PTT, RPR, urinalysis; echocardiogram; transcranial Doppler for carotid and vertebrobasilar territories, 24-hour Holter monitor.

Differential Diagnosis: Intracranial hemorrhage, seizure disorder, migraine, primary or metastatic brain neoplasm, Bell's palsy, subdural/epidural hematoma, hypertensive encephalopathy, toxins, factitious stroke.

General Measures: Head of bed at 20 degrees, turn q2h when awake, range of motion exercises qid, Foley catheter, eggcrate mattress, sheepskin blanket, heal & elbow pads. Guaiac stools.

Treatment: Supportive measures such as appropriate DVT prophylaxis, NPO, bed rest, judicious BP control (keep MAP generally 90 to 100 mmHg), physical/occupational/speech therapy.

COMPLETED ISCHEMIC STROKE:

-Aspirin enteric coated 325 mg PO qd (non-hemorrhagic strokes).

TRANSIENT ISCHEMIC ATTACK

-Determine the of source of emboli.

-Aspirin 325 mg PO qd **OR**

-Ticlopidine (Ticlid) 250 mg PO bid **OR**

-Heparin (accelerating, recurrent TIA's; cardiogenic, or vertebrobasilar)(no bolus) 700-800 U/hr (12 U/Kg/hr) IV infusion (25,000 U in 500 mL D5W); adjust q6-12h until PTT 1.2-1.4 x control (multiple TIA's cardio embolism, brainstem, evolving stroke, not large infarcts because of risk of hemorrhage).

-Warfarin (Coumadin) 5.0-7.5 mg PO qd x 3d, then 2-4 mg PO qd. Maintain PT 1.2-1.3 x control or INR 2.0-2.5.; continue warfarin for patients with evidence of cardiogenic or vertebrobasilar sources.

INTRACRANIAL HEMORRHAGE
INTRAPARENCHYMAL

Presentation: Symptoms frequently abrupt in onset including severe headache, coma, seizure, nausea/vomiting, hemiparesis, ataxia, nystagmus.

Diagnosis:

A. Noncontrast head CT (most commonly located in the putamen, subcortical white matter, thalamus, pons, cerebellum in order of occurrence).

B. Lumbar puncture may be contraindicated because of herniation risk;

C. Angiography may be indicated if surgery is planned.

D. PT/PTT, CBC

Differential Diagnosis: Subdural/epidural hematoma, seizure, neoplasm (especially glioblastoma), toxins (cocaine, amphetamine), disseminated intravascular coagulation.

Treatment:

A. **Indications for Surgery:** Hemorrhage into the cerebellum, acceleratins lobe, or if hydrocephalus.

B. **Seizure Management:** Phenytoin 15-20 mg/kg IV load NS at maximum rate of 50 mg/min, then 100 mg IVP q8h or 200 mg IVP q12h, monitor levels..

C. **Intracranial Hypertension:** Mechanical hyperventilation is most beneficial; consider steroids; shunting for hydrocephalus; mannitol 1 gm/kg followed by 0.25 gm/kg prn (monitor electrolytes). Consider pentobarbital coma (see page 124).

D. **Blood Pressure Control:** Avoid hypotension, keep mean arterial blood pressure between 90-100 mmHg with labetalol 20-80 mg IVP q15min or 0.5-2.0 mg/min IV infusion.

E. General measures include DVT prophylaxis with pneumatic compression stockings, bed rest, acetaminophen, stool softeners, neurology/neurosurgery consultation, physical/occupational/speech therapy.

SUBARACHNOID HEMORRHAGE

Saccular Aneurysm Rupture

Presentation: "Worst" headache ever, nausea/vomiting, mydriasis, visual field defects, hemiparesis, coma. Fundoscopy may show retinal hemorrhages/papilledema.

Diagnosis:
1. Noncontrast head CT scan should be done.
2. If CT is nondiagnostic, a lumbar puncture is mandatory to exclude hemorrhage. Look for xanthochromia, uniform cell count.
3. Cerebral arteriography if surgery is being considered.

Labs: CBC, SMA 12, lipid profile, INR/PTT, VDRL, ESR, UA. CXR, ECG.

Differential Diagnosis: Intracerebral hemorrhage, subdural/epidural hematoma.

Treatment:
1. Airway control with intubation as necessary.
2. Neurosurgical consult.
   Surgical Indications: High rate of rebleeding, ventricular drainage, hydrocephalus unresponsive to diuresis.
3. Avoid stimulation; keep room dark and quiet; no rectal exam or lumbar puncture; consider cerebral angiography.
4. **Vasospasm Prevention:** Nimodipine (Nimotop) 60 mg PO or via NG tube q4h x 21 days, start as soon as possible (within 96 hours).
5. Stool softeners, DVT prophylaxis with pneumatic compression stockings.
6. **Blood Pressure Control:**
   -Avoid hypotension, keep MAP 90-100 mmHg
   -Labetalol (Normodyne) 20-80 mg IV over 2 min, q10-15 min, or infuse 0.5-2.0 mg/min **OR**

-Nitroprusside sodium, 0.1-10.0 µg/kg/min (50-200 mg/250 mL NS), titrate **OR**

-Propranolol 1-3 mg IV q6h or 10-60 mg PO qid, titrate to BP <160/90, avoid if hypotensive or bradycardic

7. **Seizure Management:**
   -Phenytoin (if seizure) IV load 15-20 mg/kg IV in NS (infuse at max 50 mg/min), then 300 mg IV qAM or 200 mg q12h(4-6 mg/kg/d).

8. **Hydrocephalus:** Use of mannitol 1 gm/kg, then 0.25 gm/kg IV qid-monitor electrolytes. Dexamethasone 10 mg IV followed by 4 mg q6h.

9. **Symptomatic Medications:**
   -Codeine 15 to 60 mg q4-6h-without excessive sedation to mask mental status.
   -Ranitidine (Zantac) 50 mg IV q6-8h or 150 mg PO bid **OR**
   -Cimetidine (Tagamet) 300 mg IV q6-8h or 300 mg PO tid-qid.
   -Acetaminophen 325 mg 1-2 tabs PR q4-6h prn temp > 100.

INCREASED INTRACRANIAL PRESSURE

Presentation: Headache, lethargy; blurring of vision leading to gradual blindness in chronic cases, lethargy, diplopia, vomiting.

Diagnosis: CT/MRI of head; intracranial pressure monitor; lumbar puncture is contraindicated.

Management:

1. **Neurosurgical Evaluation.**
2. **Hyperventilation:** Short long term benefit may be life saving in cases of herniation; administer nontoxic levels of oxygen; maintain mild respiratory alkalosis-$PaCO_2$ 25-30 mmHg.
3. **Osmotic Diuresis:** Mannitol 1 gm/kg followed by 0.25 gm/kg IV qid; avoid hyperosmolarity-keep serum osmolarity less than 315 mOsm/L; initial effects occurs in less than 60 minutes.
4. **Steroids:** Dexamethasone (anti-edema effect is most benificial in presence of tumors); 10 mg initially followed by 4 mg q6h IV/PO; check glucose; avoid long term therapy.
5. Restrict fluids to ½ maintenance, isotonic fluids. Head of bed at 30 degrees, head midline.
6. Neuromuscular blockade to decrease intrathoracic pressure resulting in decrease cerebral blood flow. Concurrent use of amnesic and/or sedative agents is mandatory.
7. Pentobarbital (barbiturate coma) 7.5 mg/kg/h IV for 3h, then 2-3 mg/kg/h IV infusion, maintain ICP < 15 mmHg, CPP > 60 mmHg, MAP > 70 mmHg, and pentobarbital level of 25-40 mg/L. Use

barbiturate coma if hyperventilation, osmotic diuresis and neuromuscular blockade clinically are inadequate.

SEIZURE & STATUS EPILEPTICUS

<u>Diagnosis:</u> Obtain description of seizure from witness
EEG: May be normal in interictal period or continuous spiking with generalized seizures.
EKG; CT of head when stable (hemorrhage, tumor); lumbar puncture.

Differential Diagnosis: Toxins (drugs, withdrawal), hypoglycemia, hypernatremia or hyponatremia, hypocalcemia; hypomagnesemia, anoxia, encephalopathy (uremic or hepatic), bacterial or viral meningitis or encephalitis; tumors, cerebrovascular accident, shivering, sepsis, factitious seizure.

Management of Status Epilepticus:

1. Maintain airway; intubate as necessary; monitor cardiopulmonary status.
2. Intravenous line with normal saline; draw labs; administer thiamine 50 mg IV, D50 50 cc.
3. Administer lorazepam 0.1 mg/kg IV bolus.
4. Immediately follow with phenytoin 20 mg/kg IV load at 50 mg/min. May give phenytoin boluses at 5 mg/kg (max 30 mg/kg).
5. If seizing persists, give phenobarbital 15-20 mg/kg IV at 100 mg/min. Intubate for airway protection.
6. **Management of Persistent Seizures:**
   a. Coma induction with pentobarbital at 5-10 mg/kg IV load, followed by maintenance infusion of 1.0 mg/kg/hr. Continuous EEG-monitor for burst suppression.
   b. Stop pentobarbital at 12 hours and reassess (contraindications: pregnancy, porphyria, lack of established airway). Anticonvulsant pentobarbital level is 5-10 mg/L.
7. **Labs:** CBC, glucose, electrolytes, Mg, calcium, phosphate, check drug levels, blood alcohol, toxicology screen, VDRL, ABG, anticonvulsant levels. UA, drug screen. MRI with & without gadolinium, CT; EEG with hyperventilation, photic stimulation; CXR, ECG, lumbar puncture (see page 123).

MYASTHENIA GRAVIS

Presentation: Muscle fatigue, respiratory distress (vital capacity < 20 cc/kg). Myasthenia gravis may present as failure of extubation after anesthesia with neuromuscular blockers.

Diagnosis: Assess strength; review drugs (aminoglycosides, clindamycin, tetracycline, beta-adrenergic blockers, calcium-channel blockers, furosemide, lidocaine, phenytoin, oral contraceptives, neuromuscular blocking agents, Type 1A antiarrhythmics).

Tensilon test: Test dose of 2 mg IV and monitor for cholinergic crisis, then administer remaining 8 mg.

EMG (decreasing potential amplitude following exercise); anti-acetylcholine receptor antibodies; CT chest (thymoma); electrolytes, calcium, magnesium, phosphorus, thyroid studies, CBC with differential.

Differential Diagnosis: Guillain-Barré' Syndrome (absent reflexes), hypothyroidism, Bell's palsy, botulism toxin.

Management:

1. Monitor respiratory status through forced vital capacity (FVC) and maximum inspiratory pressure (MIP). FVC less than 20 cc/kg or MIP greater than -20 cm H20 reflects impending respiratory failure (may need immediate/elective intubation).

2. Treat infection and hypothyroidism; avoid incentive spirometry, neuromuscular blocking agents and other medications which may accentuate disease; allow patient to rest.

3. Titrate cholinesterase inhibitors to optimum dose and monitor FVC and MIP.

4. After anticholinesterase therapy and immunosuppression achieves adequate muscle strength, the patient should be weaned from mechanical ventilation, provided that the vital capacity remains >15 mL/kg and maximum sustainable expired pressure remains >40 cm H20.

Drug Therapy for Myasthenia Gravis:

A. **Cholinesterase Inhibitors:**

-Pyridostigmine (Mestinon) 30-180 mg PO/IV q3-6h with food, max dose 120 mg PO q3-4h; [syrup, 60 mg tab]; sustained release tablets 180-540 mg PO qd-bid (Timespans 180 mg tabs).

-Ambenonium chloride (Mytelase caplets) 5-25 mg PO tid-qid.

-Neostigmine 15 mg IM/PO q4h.

B. **Immunosuppressive Agents:**

-Corticosteroids are mainstay and once response is attained, alternate day dosing followed by maintenance therapy may be possible; azathioprine may be used as a steroid-sparing agent.

-Prednisone 30-60 mg PO qd.

-Methylprednisolone sodium succinate 2 g IV Q5 days.

-Azathioprine 2.5-3.0 mg/kg/d PO in 3-6 divided doses. Doses may be tapered to maintenance dose of 100 mg/d after maximal response has been achieved.

-Plasmapheresis with replacement solution consisting of mixture of albumin, dextran, and glucose-Ringer's solution combined with gammaglobulins or fresh frozen plasma, albumin alone or purified protein fraction.

-Intravenous immune globin 400 mg/kg/d for 5 days.

C. **Plasmapheresis:** 50 cc/kg exchanges during three to five sessions over 48 hours; need to initiate long term therapy; monitor cardiovascular status.

D. **Thymectomy:**
   1. Resolve acute crisis before the elective surgical procedure.
   2. Thymectomy is indicated for patients with thymoma; patients 15-40 years old with progressive weakness with severe generalized active disease <3-5 years duration.

GUILLAIN-BARRÉ SYNDROME

I. **Presentation:**
   A. Ascending weakness following "flu-like" illness;
   B. May follow immunization with live/attenuated virus, or diarrhea from Campylobacter jejuni; Epstein-Barr, or herpes simplex virus.
   C. Presents initially with hand and foot dysesthesia, followed by respiratory failure, ophthalmoplegia, areflexia, ataxia.

II. **Diagnosis:**
   A. Symmetric weakness with loss of deep tendon reflexes; mild or severe sensory loss; lumbar puncture (usually high protein, normal glucose);
   B. EMG with nerve conduction studies (proximal slowing with evidence of axonal loss).
   C. Electrolytes may show syndrome of inappropriate antidiuretic hormone (SIADH).
   D. IgM titers for Epstein-Barr and cytomegalovirus and HIV antibody screening.

III. **Differential Diagnosis:** Myasthenia gravis, dermatomyositis, poliomyelitis, toxic neuropathy, periodic paralysis, botulism, acute intermittent porphyria, amyotrophic lateral sclerosis, organophosphate poisoning.

IV. **Treatment:**
   A. Monitor respiratory status through forced vital capacity (FVC) and maximum inspiratory pressure (MIP); FVC less than 20 cc/kg or MIP

greater than -20 cm H20 reflects impending respiratory failure (may need immediate/elective intubation).

B. DVT prophylaxis; physiotherapy for paralyzed limbs; foam mattress to reduce risk of pressure sores, stress-induced ulcer prophylaxis.

C. **Autonomic Dysfunction:** continuous monitoring; fluids for hypotension and alpha-adrenergic blocking agents for hypertension.

D. **Plasmapheresis:**

1. Indicated for patients eminent paresis, respiratory failure, or dysphagia; exchange 250 cc/kg over 7 to 14 days; may need to repeat with recurrence.

2. Plasmapheresis has minimal impact on removal of salicylate, prednisolone, tobramycin, digoxin, digitoxin, phenytoin, and phenobarbital.

References

Drachman DA. *Approach to neurologic problems in the intensive care unit.*In: Rippe RS, Alpert JS, Fink MP. Intensive Care Medicine. 2nd ed. Boston: Little, Brown and Company, 1991;1543-1545.

Smith MC, Bleck TP. *Techniques for evaluating the cause of coma.* Journ Crit III 2(12):51-57, 1987.

Rothrock JF, Hart RG. *Antithrombotic therapy in cerebrovascular disease.* Ann Intern Med 115:885-895, 1991.

Solomon RA, Fink ME. *Current strategies for the management of aneurysmal subarachnoid hemorrhage.* Arch Neurol 44:769-774, 1987.

Phillips C. *Status epilepticus* In: Rippe RS, Alpert JS, Fink MP. Intensive Care Medicine. 2nd ed. Boston: Little, Brown and Company, 1991;1564-1569.

Aminoff MJ, Simon RP. *Status epilepticus.* Am J Med 69:657-665, 1980.

Chad DA. *Guillain-Barre' Syndrome* In: Rippe RS, Alpert JS, Fink MP. Intensive Care Medicine. 2nd ed. Boston: Little, Brown and Company, 1991;1591-1595.

Long RR. *Myasthenia gravis in the Intensive care unit.* In: Rippe RS, Alpert JS, Fink MP. Intensive Care Medicine. 2nd ed. Boston: Little, Brown and Company,1596-1600.

ENDOCRINOLOGY

By Salman J Naqvi M.D., M.Sc.

ADRENAL CRISIS

General Measures: Obtain a careful history for medications associated with hypoaldosteronism.

Labs: Serum cortisol, SMA 12, CBC, PPD, anti-adrenal antibodies, thyroid panel, aldosterone, ACTH. Free urinary cortisol, UA. ECG, CXR, CT/MRI of abdomen.

Treatment:

A. **Correction of Hypovolemia:**
   - -2-4 L D5NS at 500-1000 mL/h, first 8-12 hours, then 200-300 mL/h. Watch for signs of fluid overload. Monitor I&O and daily weight.

B. **Correction of Glucocorticoid Deficiency:**
   - -Dexamethasone 4 mg IV or IM q12h in urgent setting (will not interfere with cortisol assays), then 1 mg IV or PO qAM **OR**
   - -Hydrocortisone 200 mg IV loading, then 100 mg IV q8h, then 20 mg PO qAM & 10 mg PO qPM, double dose during stress **OR**
   - -Prednisone 5 mg PO qAM & 2.5 mg PO qPM **OR**
   - -Cortisone acetate 25 mg PO qAM, 12.5 mg qPM

C. **Correction of Hyperkalemia:**
   - -Mineralocorticoid therapy should be used if fluids and hydrocortisone do not correct hyponatremia and hyperkalemia.
   - -Fludrocortisone (Florinef) 0.1-0.2 mg PO qd. **OR**
   - -Desoxycorticosterone acetate (DOCA, Percorten) 5-10 mg IM.

D. **Correct Precipitating Factors.**

E. **ACTH Stimulation Test:**

Procedure:
   - (a) Draw blood for baseline serum cortisol, aldosterone and ACTH.
   - (b) Inject 0.25 mg Cosyntropin IV or IM. For IV use, dilute Cosyntropin in 2-5 mL NaCl 0.9% and inject over 2 minutes.

   Obtain repeat samples for cortisol and aldosterone 30 and 60 minutes after injection of Cosyntropin.

Interpretation:
   1. Normal adrenal function is indicated by a cortisol level of 20 mcg/dL or more at any time during the test, including before injection, or an increment of 6 mcg/dL above the baseline.
   2. To differentiate primary from seconary adrenal insufficiency. Cosyntropin is infused at a rate of 2 U/h for 24 h. In normal subjects, 17-hydroxysteroid excretion is increased by 25 mg/d, and plasma cortisol levels by >40 mcg/dL. In secondary disease, the maximal

increase in urinary 17-hydroxysteroid is 3-20 mg/d, and the plasma cortisol ranges from I0-40 mcg/dL. Pts with primary disease have smaller responses.

DIABETIC KETOACIDOSIS

Labs: Fingerstick glucose q1-6h. SMA 7 & ketones q4-6h until anion gap and ketones negative. SMA 12, amylase, lipase, HbA1C, phosphate, CBC, Mg, calcium, ABG, blood and sputum C&S x 2. Consider cardiac enzymes. UA C&S, urine protein, consider serum pregnancy test. CXR, ECG.

IV Fluids:
0.5-5 L NS over 1-5h (≥16 gauge), infuse at 400-1000 mL/h until hemodynamically stable, then change to 0.45% saline at 150-400 cc/hr; keep urine output > 30-60 mL/h.

Add KCL when no ECG signs of hyperkalemia (peaked T) & urine output adequate, serum K+ ≤ 5.8 mEq/L.

    Concentration.......20-40 mEq KCL/L

    Rate.....................10-40 mEq KCL/hr

May use K phosphate, 20-40 mEq/L, in place of KCL if low phosphate.

Change to **D5** 0.45% saline with 20-40 mEq KCL or K phosphate per liter when blood glucose 250-300.

Treatment:
-Oxygen at 2-5 L/min by NC.

-Insulin Regular (Humulin) 7-10 units (0.1 U/kg) IV bolus, then 7-10 U/h IV infusion (0.1 U/kg/h) (50 U in 250 mL of 0.9% saline at 35 mL/hr) (flush IV tubing with 20 mL of insulin sln before starting infusion). Adjust insulin infusion to decrease serum glucose by 100 mg/dL or less per hour.

-After 2 hr of therapy, if bicarbonate level not rising and anion gap not falling, double insulin infusion rate; when bicarbonate level >16 mEq/L and anion gap <16 mEq/L, decrease insulin infusion rate by half

-When the glucose level reaches 250 mg/dL, 5% dextrose should be added to the replacement fluids with KCL 20-40 mEq/L.

-Use 10% glucose at 50-100 mL/h if anion gap still present, & serum glucose <100 mg/dL while on insulin infusion.

-Change to subcutaneous insulin when anion gap cleared; discontinue insulin drip only 1-2h after subcutaneous dose.

NONKETOTIC HYPEROSMOLAR SYNDROME

Labs: Fingerstick glucose q1-6h. Osmolality. SMA 12, amylase, lipase, calcium, phosphate, ketones, HbA1C, CBC, blood and sputum C&S x 2. Cardiac enzymes. UA, urine C&S, thyroid panel. CXR, ECG.

IV Fluids:
1-5 L NS over 1-6h (≥ 16 gauge IV catheter) until no longer hypovolemic, then give 0.45% saline at 200-300 cc/hr. Maintain urine output ≥ 50 mL/h.
Add 20-40 mEq/L KCL when urine output adequate.

Treatment:
-Insulin Regular 3-5 U/h IV infusion (50 U in 250 mL of 0.9% saline at 15-25 mL/hr).
-Ranitidine (Zantac) 50 mg IV q6-8h or 150 mg PO bid.

THYROTOXICOSIS & HYPERTHYROIDISM
(THYROID STORM)

Labs: CBC, SMA 7&12; sensitive TSH, free T4. UA. CXR PA & LAT, ECG. Endocrine consult.

Treatment of Thyrotoxicosis & Hyperthyroidism:
-Cooling blanket prn temp >39°C. In refractory cases of hyperthermia, give chlorpromazine, 25-50 mg PO or IM q6h.
-Glucose IV to prevent or correct hypoglycemia.
-Propylthiouracil 1,000 mg PO or via nasogastric tube, then 150-300 mg PO q6h; usual maintenance dose 50 mg PO tid **OR**
-Methimazole (Tapazole) 30-60 mg PO, then maintenance of 5-10 mg PO q8h; max 60 mg/day **AND**
-Potassium iodine (SSKI) 5-10 drops PO q8h, 1h after propylthiouracil **AND**
-Dexamethasone 1-2 mg IV or PO q6h (in extreme cases in which hypotension is present) **AND**
-Propranolol 40-80 mg PO q6h or 0.5-1 mg/min, max 2-10 mg IV q3-4h.
-Acetaminophen 325 mg 1-2 tabs PO q4-6h prn temp >38°C.
-Lorazepam (Ativan) 1-2 mg IV/IM/PO q4-8h prn anxiety.

MYXEDEMA COMA & HYPOTHYROIDISM

Labs: CBC, SMA 12, blood culture x 2, TSH. Cardiac enzymes, cholesterol. UA. ECG, endocrine consult.

Treatment of Myxedema Coma & Hypothyroidism:

-Triple blankets prn temp <36°C, I&O, aspiration precautions.

-Volume replacement with NS at 200-300 cc/h & vasopressors if hypotensive. Correct hypoglycemia with 50% dextrose.

-Levothyroxine (Synthroid, T4, L-thyroxine) 200-500 mcg IV over 2-4 min, then 100-200 mcg PO or IV qd **OR** in stable patient, begin with 25-50 µg PO qd, increase by 25-50 µg PO qd at 2-3 week intervals until 50-200 mcg/d (1.7 µg/kg/d) **OR**

-Liothyronine (Cytomel, T3) 50-100 mcg PO, then 12.5-25 mcg PO bid-qid **OR**

-Hydrocortisone 100 mg IV loading, then 50-100 mg IV q8h.

REFERENCES

Adrenal:
Burke CW: Adrenocortical insufficiency. Clin Endocrinol Metab. 14:947, 1985.
May ME, Carey RM: Rapid adrenocorticotropic hormone test in practice. Am J Med, 79:679, 1985.
Williams Text Book of Endocrinology (8th Edition), 1992.
Vallotton MB: Endocrine emergencies. Disorder of the adrenal cortex. Baillieres Clin Endo and Metab, Jan 6(1):41, 1992.
Diabetes:
Berger W, Keller U: Treatment of diabetic ketoacidosis and non-ketotic hyperosmolar diabetic coma. Baillieres Clin Endo and Metab, Jan, 6(1):1, 1992.
Cefalu WT: Diabetic ketoacidosis. Critical Care Clinics, Jan7(1):89, 1991.
Israel RS: Diabetic ketoacidosis. Emerg Med Clin of North Am, Nov, 74):859, 1989.
Thyroid:
Gavin LA: Thyroid crises. Medical Clinics of North America 75:179, 1991.
Holvey D N, Goodner C J, Nicoloff J T, et al: Treatment of myxedema coma with intravenous thyroxine. Arch Intern Med 113:139,1964.
Hylander B, Rosenquist U: Treatment of myxedema coma-factors associated with fatal outcome. Acta Endocrinol 108:65,1985.
Roth RN, McAuliffe MJ: Hyperthyroidism and thyroid storm. Emerg Med Clin North Am 7:873, 1989.

NEPHROLOGY

By Kirk Voelker, MD

ACUTE RENAL FAILURE

CAUSES OF ACUTE RENAL FAILURE:

Prenal: Hypovolemia (dehydration, blood loss), intravascular hypovolemia (cirrhosis, nephrotic syndrome), poor perfusion.

Postrenal: Neurogenic bladder, prostatic hypertrophy, kidney/bladder stones, pelvic tumors, peritoneal fibrosis, etc.

Intrinsic Renal Disease:

Acute Interstitial Nephritis: Antibiotics (beta-lactam antibiotics, sulfonamides, tetracycline, rifampin, ethambutol), Diuretics (furosemide, thiazides), NSAID's; captopril, allopurinol, alpha-methyldopa.

Acute Tubular Necrosis: Nephrotoxins (drugs, contrast dye, aminoglycosides, myoglobin, myeloma), ischemia(hypotensive event, arterial thrombosis), embolic disease (atheroembolic after angiographic procedure, cardiogenic emboli, fat emboli), vasculitis (Goodpasture's, SLE), immune complex disease (post infectious, SLE, endocarditis)

Other: Hepato-renal, worsening of chronic renal failure, glomerulonephritis.

EVALUATION:

Labs: CBC, ABG, SMA 7 & 12, Mg, phosphate, calcium, uric acid, lipid panel. ESR, PT/PTT, ANA, rheumatoid, anti-glomerular basement membrane, VDRL, HEPATITIS B SURFACE ANTIGEN, serum protein electrophoresis, erythropoietin. UA with micro, urine Gram stain, C&S; urine electrolytes, creatinine.

TREATMENT:

Prerenal:

Hypovolemia: Replace volume with normal saline infusions.

Cirrhosis, Nephrotic Syndrome: Improve perfusion, colloid, spironolactone.

Poor Perfusion: Administer inotropes, provide afterload reduction.

Post Renal: Remove obstruction or place a stent to decompress kidney.

Intrinsic Renal Disease:

1. Correct underlying disorder, remove all nephrotoxic drugs, when patient becomes euvolemic.

2. **Loop Diuretics:** Lasix 40 mg IV, double every 30 min. If no response after 300 mg then give metolazone 5-10 mg PO, and repeat Lasix 300 mg IV thirty minutes later. Once an effective dose found continue q8 hrs. Diuretics may convert oliguric to non-oliguric renal

failure as well as decrease the metabolic demand of the failing kidney; high doses of Lasix may cause ototoxicity.

3. **Renal Dose Dopamine** (2-3 mcg/kg/min): Improve renal blood flow
4. **Mannitol** 12.5-25 mg IV q8; use cautiously if oliguria; contraindicated if hypovolemia.

General Measures: Avoid magnesium containing antacids, salt substitutes, NSAIDS, & other nephrotoxins. Avoid phosphates or potassium unless depleted.

Diet: Renal diet of high biologic value protein of 0.6 to 0.8 g/kg, sodium 2 g, potassium 1 mEq/kg, and at least 35 kcal/kg of nonprotein calories .

HYPOCALCEMIA

Clinical Manifestations of Hypocalcemia: Hypotension, bradycardia, arrhythmias, ECG (QT, T's), bronchospasm, apnea, laryngeal spasm, tetany, seizures, weakness, psychosis, confusion.

Clinical Evaluation of Hypocalcemia:

I. **Check ionized calcium and repeat 2 times, if low then:**
   A. Rule out Renal Failure, history of parathyroid/thyroid deficiency, surgery or trauma, nephrotic syndrome.
   B. **Exclude Drug-related Hypocalcemia:** Aminoglycosides, calcitonin, cisplatin, diphosphonates, ethylene glycol, heparin, loop diuretics, magnesium, phenobarbital, phenytoin, phosphates.

II. **Check Serum Magnesium:**
   A. If High, consider: Suppression of PTH by hypermagnesemia.
   B. If Low, consider: Aminoglycosides, Amphotericin B, alcoholism, pancreatitis.

III. **Check Serum Phosphate:**
   A. If High, consider: Renal insufficiency, excess phosphate intake, rhabdomyolysis.

IV. **Check Parathyroid Hormone Level:**
   A. If Low, consider: Hypoparathyroidism, sepsis, pancreatitis, hypermagnesemia.
   B. If Normal, consider: Malignancy, increased osteoblastic activity.

V. **Check 25-hydroxy Vitamin D_3:**
   A. If Low, consider: Vitamin D deficiency, liver disease, malabsorption.

VI. **Check 1,25-hydroxy Vitamin D_3**
   A. If Low, consider: Renal hydroxylase deficiency.
   B. If Normal or High, consider: peripheral resistance to parathyroid hormone.

<u>**Treatment of HYPOcalcemia:**</u>
Symptomatic HYPOcalcemia:

-Calcium chloride, 10% (270 mg calcium/10 mL vial) give 5-10 mL slowly over 5-10 min or dilute in 50-100 mL of D5 & infuse over 20 min, repeat q1-2h if symptomatic or q6-12h if asymptomatic <u>**OR**</u> infuse 10 mL of 10% calcium chloride in 500 mL NS over 8h. Maintain total serum calcium at 7-8 mg/dL; correct hyperphosphatemia before hypocalcemia <u>**OR**</u>

-Calcium gluconate, 20 mL of 10% solution IV (2 vials)(90 mg elemental calcium/10 mL vial) infused over 10-15 min, repeat q1-2h if symptomatic or q6-12h if asymptomatic <u>**OR**</u> infuse 1 vial in 500 mL of NS IV over 8h.

HYPERCALCEMIA

Clinical Manifestations of Hypercalcemia: Weakness, atrophy, hyporeflexia, neuropsychiatric changes, pancreatitis, osteopenia, ECG changes (QT shortening, heart block, arrhythmias).

Clinical Evaluation of Hypercalcemia:

A. Rule out Drugs (calcium, thiazides, lithium, vitamin A & D)

B. Rule out Milk-Alkali Syndrome

C. Rule out Renal disease (CRI, post ATN, transplant)

D. Rule out Familial Syndrome (FHH, MEN I, MEN II)

E. Rule out Adrenal insufficiency, hyperthyroidism

F. Rule out Malignancy, AIDS

G. Rule out Phosphorus depletion syndrome, immobilization

H. Low Urine Calcium- FHH, hypothyroidism, lithium, thiazides, Bartter's syndrome, milk-alkali, adrenal insufficiency

I. High PTH- Hyperparathyroidism

Treatment of HYPERcalcemia:

GENERAL- Treat underlying disorder, discontinue offending drugs, hydrate and correct electrolytes, restrict calcium intake, maintain phosphorus intake.

Increase Calcium Excretion:

-1-4 L of 0.9 % saline at 150-600 cc/h IV until no longer hypotensive <u>**THEN**</u>

-Saline diuresis 0.9% or 0.45% saline infused at 300-600 cc/h to replace urine loss; maintain urine output at 200-300 cc/hr, dialysis if needed <u>**AND**</u>

-Furosemide 20-40 mg IV q2-12h. Maintain urine output of 200-500 mL/h; monitor I&O q4h; closely monitor patient weight and serum sodium, potassium, magnesium; measure and replace urine Mg & K+ losses (empiric replacement: magnesium 15 mg/h & 10-30 mEq K+/h, if renal function normal).

Decrease Bone Resorption:
- -Salmon calcitonin 4 IU/kg SQ or IM q12-24h, max 8 IU/kg IM q6h. Skin test with 0.1 mL of sln (10 IU/mL) intradermally first.
- -Etidronate disodium (Didronel) 7.5 mg/Kg/day in NS 200 mLs IV over 2h qd x 3-7 days.
- -Mithramycin (Mithracin) 25 mcg/Kg/ day x 3-4 days (D5W or NS 1000 mLs over 4-6 h). Use in hypercalcemia associated with malignancy unresponsive to other measures.
- -Hydrocortisone (bone metastasis), 5 mg/kg IV q8h, then prednisone 40-100 mg PO qd.

Calcium Chelators:
- -Neutral phosphate (Nutra-Phos), 2-3 capsules (250 mg phosphate/capsule) PO tid-qid **OR** Phospho-Soda, 5 mL (645 mg phosphorus) PO tid-qid. Maintain phosphate 4-5 mg/dL & calcium-phosphate product <70.
- -EDTA 10-50 mg/kg over 4 hrs.

HYPERKALEMIA

Signs & Symptoms: Paresthesias, weakness, paralysis, confusion, arrhythmias, heart block, ECG changes (peaked T waves, small P waves, prolonged PR, wide QRS)

Differential Diagnosis of Hyperkalemia:
- A. **Exogenous K Intake**: K supplementation, stored blood, drugs (potassium salts of penicillin).
- B. **Decreased Excretion:** Renal insufficiency.
- C. **Cellular Shift:** Acidosis, catabolism, rhabdomyolysis, familial hyperkalemic periodic paralysis, drugs.
- D. **Mineralocorticoid Deficiency**: Addison's disease, hyporeninemic hypoaldosteronism.
- E. **AIDS**: Renal failure, CMV/TB adrenalitis, trimethoprim
- F. **Pseudohyperkalemia**: Thrombocytosis (>700 k), hemolysis, leukocytosis (>200,000) Drugs:(NSAID's, ACE-inhibitors, B-blockers, digoxin, K-sparing diuretics)

<u>Labs:</u> CBC, platelets, Mg, calcium, SMA-12, lactate, ABG, renin, aldosterone. UA with micro, specific gravity, Na, K, 24h urine K, Na, creatinine, cortisol. ECG.

<u>Treatment:</u>
- -Discontinue NSAIDS, angiotensin converting enzyme inhibitors, beta-blockers, K-sparing diuretics.
- -Calcium gluconate 10% sln 10 mL IV over 2-5 min; second dose may be given in 5 min. If dig toxicity suspected, give over 30 min or omit.

-NaHCO3 44-132 mEq (1-3 amps of 7.5%) IV over 5 min (give after calcium in separate IV), repeat in 10-15 min. Followed by infusion of 2-3 amps in D5W, titrated over 2-4 h.
-Insulin 10-20 U regular in 500 mL of D10W IV over 1 hr or 10 units IV push with 1 amp 50% glucose (25 gm) over 5 min, repeat as needed.
-Furosemide 40-80 mg IV q4-6h.
-Kayexalate 15-50 gm in 100 mL of 20% sorbitol solution PO now & in 3-4h; up to 4-5 doses/d.
-Kayexalate retention enema 25-50 gm in 200 mL of 20% sorbitol; retain for 30-60 min; may use Fleet enema before.
-Albuterol (acute hyperkalemia) 10-20 mg in 3 cc NS by nebulizer.
-Consider emergent dialysis if cardiac complications or renal failure.

HYPOKALEMIA

Signs & Symptoms: impaired contractility digoxin toxicity, impaired response to pressors, weakness, cramps, respiratory failure, rhabdomyolysis hyporeflexia, weakness/paralysis, confusion, polyuria, nephrogenic DI, ileus, metabolic alkalosis.

ECG Abnormalities: Wide QRS, ST depression, block, flat T-waves, U-waves.

Labs: CBC, Mg, SMA 12, ABG, renin, aldosterone. UA with micro, Na, K. bicarb, Cl, pH, 24h urine K, Na, Creatinine. Repeat electrolytes q4h until stable. ECG, dietetics consult.

Treatment:
-KCL 10-40 mEq in 100 cc saline infused IVPB over 2 hours; or add up to 10-80 mEq to 1 liter of IV fluid and infuse over 2 hours); may combine with 30-40 mEq PO q4h in addition to IV; total dose max is generally 100-200 mEq/d (3 mEq/kg/d).

Chronic Therapy:
-KCL elixir 1-3 tablespoon qd-tid PO after meals (20 mEq/Tbsp of 10% sln).
-Micro-K 10 mEq tabs 2-3 tabs PO tid after meals (40-100 mEq/d).

Hypokalemia with metabolic acidosis:
-Potassium citrate 15-30 mL in juice qid PO after meals (1 mEq/mL).
-Potassium gluconate 15 mL in juice qid PO after meals (20 mEq/15 mL).

HYPOMAGNESEMIA

Clinical Manifestation: Nausea/vomiting, cramps, anorexia, seizures, tetany, weakness, psychosis, heart failure, angina, digoxin toxicity,

ECG Manifestations: Peaked T-waves (early), broad small T-waves(late), arrhythmias (Torsades de pointes ventricular tachycardia).

Differential Diagnosis of Hypermagnesemia:

1. **Excessive stool losses:** Inflammatory bowel disease, gastroenteritis, pancreatic insufficiency, fistulas, short bowel syndrome, ileal bypass, cholestatic liver disease.
2. **Renal wasting:** Diuretics, aminoglycosides, amphotericin B, cisplatin, calcium, hyperthyroidism, diuresis.
3. **Transcellular shifts:** Refeeding/TPN, catecholamines, ethanol withdrawal), recent blood products (citrate binds magnesium).

Labs: Magnesium, calcium, SMA 12, amylase. Urine Mg, electrolytes, 24h urine Mg, creatinine, potassium. ECG.

Diagnostic Approach to Hypomagnesemia:

1. Measure 24 hr urine magnesium.
2. If greater urine magnesium is greater than 3 mg/day then renal wasting is the likely cause.
3. If urine magnesium is less than 3 mg/day, then excess magnesium intake is the likely cause.

Treatment:

-Magnesium sulfate, 5 g in 500 mL D5W IV over 3-5 hrs, then 6-9 gm/day continue to replace over 5-7 days (reduce dose for renal insufficiency). If hypocalcemic, give MgCl2 instead of magnesium sulfate (sulfate chelates calcium). Hold dose if no patellar reflex.

-Magnesium sulfate (severe hypomagnesemia <1.0) 1-2 gm (2-4 mL of 50% sln) (8-16 mEq)) IV over 15 min **OR**

-Magnesium sulfate 1 gm (2 mL of 50% sln) IM q4-6h **OR**

-Magnesium chloride (Slow-Mag) 65-130 mg (1-2 tabs) PO tid-qid (64 mg or 5.3 mEq/tab)

-Hold digoxin until hypomagnesemia resolved; monitor calcium and potassium levels.

HYPERMAGNESEMIA

Clinical Manifestations: decreased reflexes, hypotension.

Evaluation:

1. Rule out exogenous magnesium intake in the form of antacids, parenteral nutrition, enema use.
2. Rule out Renal insufficiency, hypothyroidism, Addison's disease, lithium excess, familial hypocalcemia

Labs: Magnesium, calcium, SMA 12. Urine Mg, electrolytes, 24h urine Mg, creatinine. ECG.

Therapy: Supportive care.

-Saline diuresis 0.9% or 0.45% saline infused at 300-600 cc/h to replace urine loss.

-Furosemide 20-40 mg IV q2h. Monitor I&O and patient weigh and serum calcium, sodium, potassium, magnesium.

-Calcium gluconate (if hypocalcemic)(10% sln; 1 gm (4.6 mEq) per 10 mL amp) 1-3 ampules added to saline infusate.

-Hold all magnesium containing meds including Mg antacids.

HYPERNATREMIA

A. **Clinical Manifestations of Hypernatremia:**
   1. Clinical manifestations include signs of volume overload or volume depletion, tremulousness, irritability, ataxia, spasticity, mental confusion, seizures, and coma. Symptoms are more likely to occur with acute increases in plasma sodium.

B. **Diagnostic Approach to Hypernatremia:**
   1. **Hypernatremia with ECF Volume Depletion:**
      a. Occurs with hypotonic fluid loss, typically in patients who are unable to obtain water in the face of ongoing extrarenal losses (gastrointestinal and insensible losses).
      b. Urine volume is decreased and U_{osm} is high. Renal losses due to the presence of a diuretic or an osmotic diuresis (hyperglycemia) should be suspected if both urine volume and osmolality are high. If urine volume is high but urine osmolality is low, diabetes insipidus is the most likely cause.
   2. **Hypernatremia with ECF Volume Expansion:**
      a. Usually seen in patients receiving hypertonic saline or $NaHCO_3$.
      b. Mild hypernatremia occurs with primary hyperaldosteronism and Cushing's syndrome.

Treatment:

Hypernatremia Volume Depletion:

If volume depleted, give 0.5-3 L NS IV at over 1-3 hours until not orthostatic, then give D5W (if hyperosmolar) or D5½NS (if not hyperosmolar) IV to replace half of body water deficit over first 24h (attempt to correct sodium at 1 mEq/L/h), then remaining deficit over next 1-2 days.

Body water deficit (L) = $\dfrac{0.6(\text{weight kg})([\text{Na serum}]-140)}{140}$

Hypernatremia with ECF Volume Expansion:

-Therapy consists of removal of the excess sodium with diuretics or dialysis (if renal failure) followed by replacement of fluid losses with 5% dextrose water.

-Furosemide 40-80 mg IV or PO qd-bid.

HYPONATREMIA

Clinical Evaluation of Hyponatremia:

A. Excluded pseudohyponatremia, then determine the cause of the hyponatremia based on history, physical exam, urine osmolality, and urine sodium level. Determine if the patient is volume contracted, normal volume, or volume expanded.

B. **Classify Patients Based on Urine Osmolality:**

Low Urine Osmolality (50-180 mOsm/L): Indicates primary excessive water intake (psychogenic water drinking).

High Urine Osmolality (urine osmolality > serum osmolality):

High Urine Sodium (>40 mEq/L) and Volume Contracted: Indicates a renal source of fluid loss (excessive diuretic use, salt-wasting nephropathy, Addison's disease, osmotic diuresis).

High Urine Sodium (>40 mEq/L) and Normal Volume: Most likely due to water retention caused by a drug effect, hypothyroidism, or the syndrome of inappropriate antidiuretic hormone secretion.

Drugs that can cause water retention: Chlorpropamide (Diabinese), carbamazepine, amitriptyline, vincristine, cyclophosphamide. In SIADH, the urine sodium level is usually high, but may be low if salt-restricted diet; found in the presence of a malignant tumor or a disorder of the pulmonary or central nervous system.

Low Urine Sodium (<20 mEq/L) and Volume Contraction: Dry mucous membranes, decreased skin turgor, orthostatic hypotension. Indicates an extrarenal source of fluid loss (gastrointestinal disease, burns).

Low Urine Sodium (<20 mEq/L) and Volume-expanded, Edematous: Caused by congestive heart failure, cirrhosis with ascites, and nephrotic syndrome; effective arterial blood volume is decreased. Decreased renal perfusion causes increased reabsorption of water.

Treatment:

For each 100 mg/dL ↑ in glucose, Na+ ↓ by 1.6 mEq/L.

Hyponatremia with increased ECF & edema (Hypervolemia)(low osmolality <280, UNa <10 mMol/L: nephrosis, CHF, cirrhosis; UNa >20: acute/chronic renal failure):

-Water restrict 0.5-1.5 L/d.

-Furosemide 40-80 mg IV or PO qd (20-600 mg/d).

-If severe symptomatic hyponatremia, may need concurrent diuresis and sodium replacement. Rule out sepsis.

Hyponatremia with Isovolemia (low osmolality <280, UNa <10 mMol: water intoxication; UNa >20: SIADH, hypothyroidism, renal failure, Addison's disease, Stress, Drugs):

-Furosemide 80 mg (1 mg/kg) IV qd-bid (20-600 mg/d) **AND**

-0.9% saline with 20-40 mEq KCL/L at 65-150 cc/h (correct rate < 0.5 mEq/L/h).

-Water restrict to 500-1500 mL/d.

Hyponatremia with Hypovolemia (low osmolality <280) UNa <10 mMol/L: vomiting, diarrhea, 3rd space/respiratory/skin loss; UNa >20 mMol/L: diuretics, renal injury, RTA, adrenal insufficiency, partial obstruction, salt wasting:

If volume depleted, give 0.5-3 L of 0.9% saline at 500 cc/h until no longer orthostatic, then 0.9% saline (125 mEq/L) with 10-40 mEq KCl/L at 65-150 cc/h (determine volume as below) or 100 cc 3 % hypertonic saline over 5h.

Severe Symptomatic Hyponatremia:

-If volume depleted, give 0.5-3 L of 0.9% saline at 500 cc/h until no longer orthostatic.

-Determine vol of 3% hypertonic saline (513 mEq/L) to be infused:

$$\text{Na (mEq) deficit} = 0.6 \times (\text{wt kg}) \times (\text{desired[Na]}-\text{actual[Na]})$$

$$\frac{\text{Volume of sln (L)}}{\text{Number of hrs}} = \frac{\text{Sodium to be infused (mEq)}}{(\text{mEq/L in sln}) \times \text{Number of hrs}}$$

-Correct half of sodium deficit IV slowly over 24h to 120 mEq/L or increase by 12-20 mEq/L over 24h (1 mEq/L/h).

-Furosemide 40-80 mg IV or PO qd-bid.

-3% saline 100 cc over 4-6h repeat as needed (alternative method).

-Avoid overly rapid correction, avoid volume overload.

HYPOPHOSPHATEMIA

Clinical Manifestations: Heart failure, muscle weakness, tremor, ataxia, seizures, coma, respiratory failure, delayed weaning from ventricular, hemolysis, rhabdomyolysis.

Differential Diagnosis of Hypophosphatemia: Pregnancy, dialysis, inadequate intake. Drugs: Anabolic steroids, corticosteroids, calcitonin, antacids, diuretics, insulin, salicylates, parenteral nutrition.

Labs: Phosphate, SMA 12, LDH, Mg, Cal, albumin, GGT, CPK, uric acid, ABG, 1,25(OH)vitamin D, PTH, urine electrolytes, pH. 24h urine phosphate, creatinine, potassium, UA with micro. CXR PA & LAT, ECG.

Diagnostic Approach to Hypophosphatemia:

24 hr Urine Phosphate:

A. If 24 hour urine phosphate is less than 100 mg/day the causes include gastrointestinal losses (emesis, diarrhea, NG suction, phosphate binders, malabsorption), vitamin D deficit, refeeding, recovery from burns, alkalosis, alcoholism, DKA, ASA overdose.

B. If 24 hour urine phosphate is greater than 100 mg/day, the causes include renal losses, hyperparathyroidism, hypomagnesemia, hypokalemia, acidosis, diuresis, renal tubular defects, vitamin D deficiency.

Therapy:

Mild Hypophosphatemia:

-Na or K phosphate 0.25 mMol/Kg IV infusion at the rate of 10 mMoles/hr (NS or D5W 150-250 mLs); MR prn.

-Neutral phosphate (Nutra-Phos), 2 capsules PO bid-tid (250 mg elemental phosphorus/tab, 7 mEq Na+ & 7 mEq K+/tab)**OR**

-Phospho-Soda (129 mg phosphorus & 4.8 mEq Na+/mL) 5 mL PO bid-tid.

Severe Hypophosphatemia:

-Na or K phosphate 0.5 m Moles/Kg IV infusion at the rate of 10 mMoles/hr (NS or D5W 150-250 mLs); MR prn.

-Add potassium phosphate to IV solution in place of KCl (max 40 mEq/L infused at 100-150 mL/h). Max IV dose 7.5 mg phosphorus/kg/6-8h **OR** 2.5-5 mg elemental phosphorus/kg IV over 6-8h. Give as potassium or sodium phosphate (93 mg phos/mL & 4 mEq Na+ or K+/mL). Do not mix calcium & phosphorus in same IV.

-Follow K+ level; if hypokalemia, consider sodium phosphate supplementation.

HYPERPHOSPHATEMIA

Clinical Manifestations of Hyperphosphatemia: Hypotension, bradycardia, arrhythmias, bronchospasm, apnea, laryngeal spasm, tetany, seizures, weakness, psychosis, confusion.

Clinical Evaluation of Hyperphosphatemia:

1. **Rule out Exogenous Phosphate Administration:** Enemas, laxatives, diphosphonates vitamin D excess.

2. **Rule out Endocrine Disturbances:** Hypoparathyroidism, acromegaly, PTH resistance.

3. **Rule Out Excess Phosphate Production:** Rhabdomyolysis, sepsis, fulminant hepatic failure, severe hypothermia, hemolysis, acidosis, renal failure, chemotherapy, tumor lysis syndrome.

Labs: Phosphate, SMA 12, Mg, Cal, parathyroid hormone. 24h urine phosphate, creatinine, UA. CXR PA & LAT, ECG.

Therapy: Correct hypocalcemia, restrict dietary phosphate, saline diuresis.

Moderate Hyperphosphatemia:

-Aluminum hydroxide (Amphojel) 5-10 mL or 1-2 tablets PO ac tid **OR**

-Aluminum carbonate (Basaljel) 5-10 mL or 1-2 tablets PO ac tid **OR**

-Calcium carbonate (Oscal) (250 or 500 mg elemental calcium/tab) 1-2 gm elemental calcium PO ac tid. Keep calcium-phosphate product <70; start only if phosphate <5.5.

-Aluminum containing agents bind to unabsorbed phosphate in the GI system, thus decreasing phosphate absorption.

Severe Hyperphosphatemia:

-Volume expansion with 0.9% saline 1-3 L over 1-6h.

-Acetazolamide (Diamox) 500 mg PO or IV q6h.

-Consider dialysis.

FORMULAS

A-a gradient = $[(P_B - PH_2O) FiO_2 - PCO_2/R] - PO_2$ arterial

$\quad\quad\quad\quad = (713 \times FiO2 - pCO2/0.8) - pO2$ arterial

P_B = 760 mmHg; PH_2O = 47 mmHg ; R ≈ 0.8
normal Aa gradient <10-15 mmHg (room air)

Arterial oxygen capacity =(Hgb(gm)/100 mL) x 1.36 mL O2/gm Hgb

Arterial O2 content = 1.36(Hgb)(SaO2)+0.003(PaO2)= NL 20 vol%

O2 delivery = CO x arterial O2 content = NL 640-1000 ml O2/min

Cardiac output = HR x stroke volume

CO L/min = $\dfrac{125 \text{ ml O2/min/M}^2}{8.5\{(1.36)(Hgb)(SaO2)-(1.36)(Hgb)(SvO2)\}}$ x 100

(need to multiply by M^2 to get CO estimate for a patient. This is CI estimate)

Note: 125 is a crude estimate for normals
Normal CO = 4-6 L/min

SVR = $\dfrac{MAP-CVP}{CO_{L/min}}$ x 80 = NL 800-1200 dyne/sec/cm^2

PVR = $\dfrac{PA-PCWP}{CO_{L/min}}$ x 80 = NL 45-120 dyne/sec/cm^2

GFR ml/min = $\dfrac{(140-age) \times \text{ wt in Kg}}{72 \text{ (males) x serum Cr (mg/dl)}}$
$\quad\quad\quad\quad\quad\quad$ 85 (females) x serum Cr (mg/dl)

Creatinine clearance = $\dfrac{U \text{ Cr (mg/100 mL)} \times U \text{ vol (mL)}}{P \text{ Cr (mg/100 mL)} \times \text{time (1440 min for 24h)}}$

Normal creatinine clearance = 100-125 ml/min(males), 85-105(females)

Body water deficit (L) = $\dfrac{0.6(\text{weight kg})[\text{measured serum Na}]-140)}{140}$

Osmolality mOsm/kg = 2[Na+ K] + $\dfrac{BUN}{2.8}$ + $\dfrac{glucose}{18}$ = NL 270-290 $\dfrac{mOsm}{kg}$

Fractional excreted Na = $\dfrac{U \text{ Na/ Serum Na}}{U \text{ Cr/ Serum Cr}}$ x 100 = NL<1%

Anion Gap = Na + K-(Cl + HCO3)

For each 100 mg/dl ↑ in glucose, Na+ ↓ by 1.6 mEq/L.

Corrected$\quad\quad\quad\quad$ = measured Ca mg/dl + 0.8 x (4-albumin g/dl)
serum Ca$^+$ (mg/dl)

Ideal body weight males = 50 kg for first 5 feet of height + 2.3 kg for each
$\quad\quad$ additional inch.

Ideal body weight females = 45.5 kg for first 5 feet + 2.3 kg for each additional
$\quad\quad$ inch.

Basal energy expenditure (BEE):
  Males=66 + (13.7 x actual weight Kg) + (5 x height cm)-(6.8 x age)
  Females= 655+(9.6 x actual weight Kg)+(1.7 x height cm)-(4.7 x age)

Nitrogen Balance = Gm protein intake/6.25-urine urea nitrogen-(3-4 gm/d insensible loss)

Predicted Maximal Heart Rate = 220-age

Normal ECG Intervals (sec)

PR	0.12-0.20
QRS	0.06-0.08

Heart rate/min	**Q-T**
60	0.33-0.43
70	0.31-0.41
80	0.29-0.38
90	0.28-0.36
100	0.27-0.35

DRUG LEVELS OF COMMON MEDICATIONS

DRUG	THERAPEUTIC RANGE*
Amikacin	Peak 25-30; trough <10 mcg/ml
Amiodarone	1.0-3.0 mcg/ml
Amitriptyline	100-250 ng/ml
Carbamazepine	4-10 mcg/ml
Chloramphenicol	Peak 10-15; trough <5 mcg/ml
Desipramine	150-300 ng/ml
Digitoxin	10-30 ng/ml
Digoxin	0.8-2.0 ng/ml
Disopyramide	2-5 mcg/ml
Doxepin	75-200 ng/ml
Ethosuximide	40-100 mcg/ml
Flecainide	0.2-1.0 mcg/ml
Gentamicin	Peak 6.0-8.0; trough <2.0 mcg/ml
Imipramine	150-300 ng/ml
Lidocaine	2-5 mcg/ml
Lithium	0.5-1.4 meq/L
Mexiletine	1.0-2.0 mcg/ml
Nortriptyline	50-150 ng/ml
Phenobarbital	10-30 meq/ml
Phenytoin**	8-20 mcg/ml
Procainamide	4.0-8.0 mcg/ml
Quinidine	2.5-5.0 mcg/ml
Salicylate	15-25 mg/dl
Streptomycin	Peak 10-20; trough <5 mcg/ml
Theophylline	8-20 mcg/ml
Tocainide	4-10 mcg/ml
Valproic acid	50-100 mcg/ml
Vancomycin	Peak 30-40; trough <10 mcg/ml

* The therapeutic range of some drugs may vary depending on the reference lab used.

** Therapeutic range of phenytoin is 4-10 mcg/ml in presence of significant azotemia and/or hypoalbuminemia.

ORDER FORM

Books from Current Clinical Strategies Publishing:

Current Clinical Strategies, Practice Parameters in Medicine, Primary Care, Family Practice, and Gynecology	#___ x $16.75
Current Clinical Strategies, **PEDIATRIC** DRUG RESOURCE	#___ x $8.75
Handbook of Anesthesiology Mark Ezekiel, MD	#___ x $8.75
Manual of HIV/AIDS Therapy Laurence Peiperl, MD	#___ x $8.75
Current Clinical Strategies, MEDICINE, Paul D. Chan, MD NEW 1996 edition	#___ x $8.75
Current Clinical Strategies, GYNECOLOGY & OBSTETRICS, NEW 1995 edition	#___ x $10.75
Current Clinical Strategies, PEDIATRICS, NEW 1995 edition	#___ x $8.75
FAMILY MEDICINE, NEW 1995 edition Pediatrics, Medicine, Gynecology, Obstetrics	#___ x $26.25
DIAGNOSTIC HISTORY & PHYSICAL EXAMINATION in MEDICINE	#___ x $8.75
OUTPATIENT MEDICINE	#___ x $8.75
CRITICAL CARE MEDICINE, 1995 edition	#___ x $12.75
PSYCHIATRY	#___ x $8.75
HANDBOOK OF PSYCHIATRIC DRUG THERAPY	#___ x $8.75
Current Clinical Strategies, SURGERY	#___ x $8.75
Current Clinical Strategies, PHYSICIAN'S DRUG RESOURCE (Adult dosages)	#___ x $8.75

Shipping and Handling, add $3.00 per book $ _____

Total $ _____

Enclose the cover of your old edition, and receive $2.00 off your order when you purchase
the new edition.

Please complete reverse side.

Prices are in US dollars. Other countries, send equivalent amount in foreign check. Prices and Availability subject to change without notice.

Order by Phone: 714-965-9400 (a bill will be sent with order)

Order by Mail. Send order & check payable to:

Current Clinical Strategies Publishing
9550 Warner Ave, Suite 213
Fountain Valley, Ca USA 92708-2822

Return Address: _____

_____

_____

_____

Phone Number: (_____)_____

Comments:

We appreciate your comments about our books and software.

Suggested additions or corrections:

_____

_____

_____

_____

_____

_____

_____